Preface

Yvonne Lightner 02/02/1957- 11/05/2013

It had been a tough journey for my mother Yvonne Lightner for so many years yet she never gave in to despair or disappointment. I looked to her often in awe not just because she was my mother but, a true champion of humanity. A rare being who truly believed that every person has redeeming qualities. Even in death her aura shines as a beacon of brilliant radiance even in the most foreboding abyss of darkness. She was and will always remain as the most influential person in my life.

Scholastically, she was truly a brilliant student graduating from high school as a junior. During graduation she walked with her older sister (a senior), taking top honors at graduation. As a dedicated wife and mother she and the late Gregory T. Lightner Sr. managed to stay together until my brothers and I were adults with our own families. During the 30 years they were together the built and operated a business that would carry the family and set in motion a blueprint of sorts for me and my two siblings to follow. Both my mother and father were very committed to the communities that they loved so dearly and before each of them passed, they would leave their respective mark on the world. Yvonne as a philanthropist donated her time, money and soul to the Lupus Foundation of America. She was instrumental in educating many men & women about the symptoms of Lupus saving many from misdiagnosis. Also as she was an outspoken opponent of domestic violence and domestic abuse and she would often speak to battered men & women. Additionally, she was a writer who found comfort in sharing prayers that she and her best friend & youngest sister Cathy Trice composed daily.

One of the most impressive qualities that I admired was my mother's strength. Despite of the debilitating and crippling effects of Lupus, she was determined to have fun and engage her grandchildren. Not a day would pass that she was not taking the kids out for snacks, to the parks, or the pool. Often she keep goodies in her room and the kids would sprint off the bus with good grades in hand right to Grandma. During the summer of 2012 we had a full house, my brother Aaron's children spent the summer with us. It was a site to see; so many Lightner babies, all eight jostling for position on Grandma Yvonne... Savion, Shane, Seth and Micaila.

Time and again throughout the years, I would observe my mother remain calm in some of the most difficult situations. She had a way of compartmentalizing issue after issue, removing people who were not productive or conductive to her well-being from her life. She believed that this was the secret to happiness and longevity of life and I have learned to do the same. All that I have achieved and will achieve in the future is a testimony to her perseverance, love and determination.

DEDICATION

This book is dedicated in loving memory of: Yvonne Lightner, Mr. & Mrs. Alex McLain, Mrs. Lula Trice, Paul L Trice, Mr. Jimmie T Trice Sr., Jimmie T Trice Jr., Thomas Lightner, Gregory T Lightner Sr. and Mrs. Bernice Mills Lightner.

Also dedicated to all whom fight Lupus

and their caregivers.

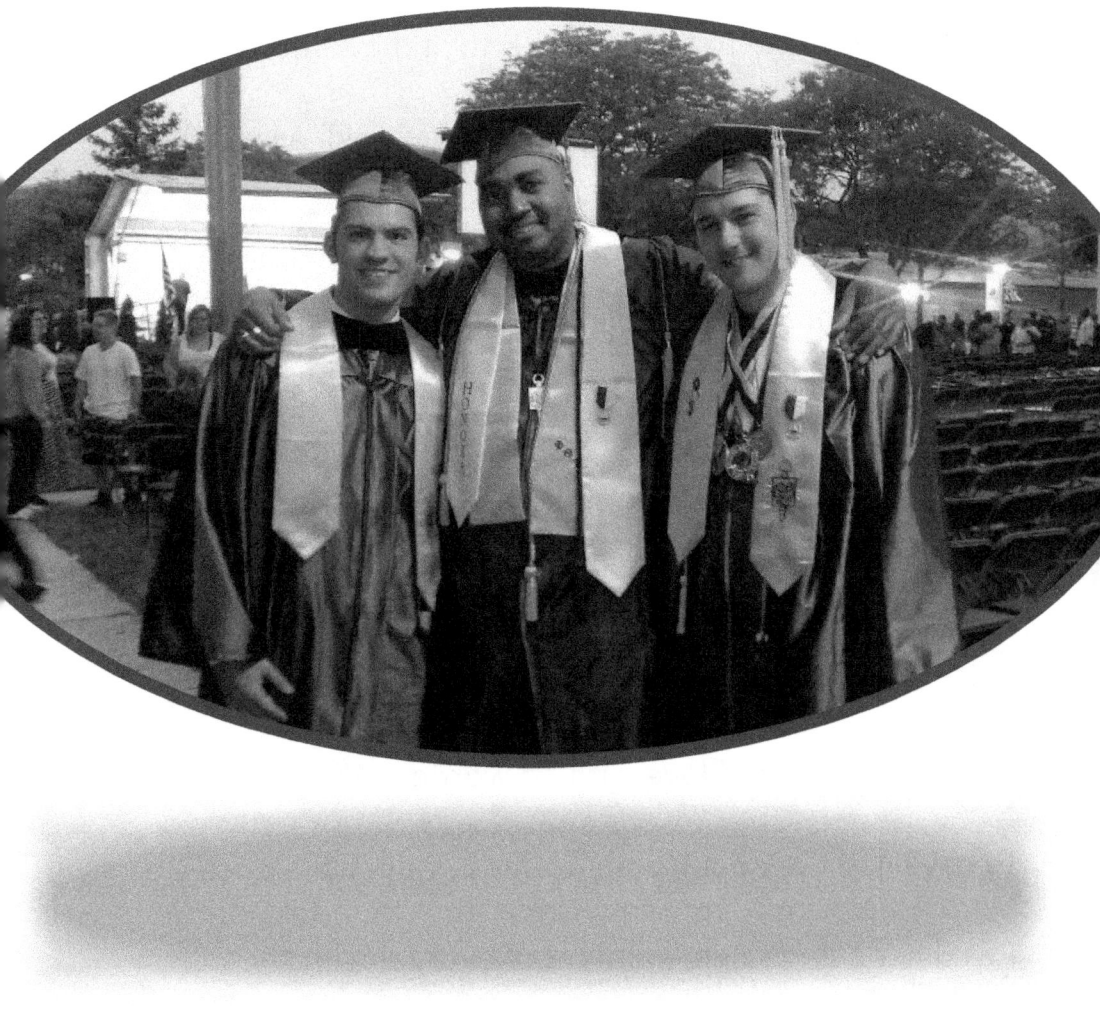

When Yvonne Lightner passed on November 5th 2013 she was finally at peace and reunited with her family who have preceded her in death. Matriarch Yvonne Lightner was able to leave this earth in the same way she lived; honored, respected, loved and revered. As we promised her so many years ago, my wife Gigi Lightner, and our children Giana, Gilina, Gevont, and Giavonna were with her every step for the last three years of her journey. She was never alone and for the first time in her life she said she felt "free". This was instrumental in her having the time to really enjoy the fruits of a most demanding labor of love with no worries. We feel blessed to have had the opportunity to show mom how much we loved her every single moment of every single day.

While we miss her smiles, long talks on the porch & infectious laughs, we are not sad nor do we despair. Mother was able to go from here knowing that the book that we worked so hard on over the last few years would be given to the world as her parting gift to those who are coping with Lupus or may have Lupus & their caregivers. May her voice fill you with joy and understanding........

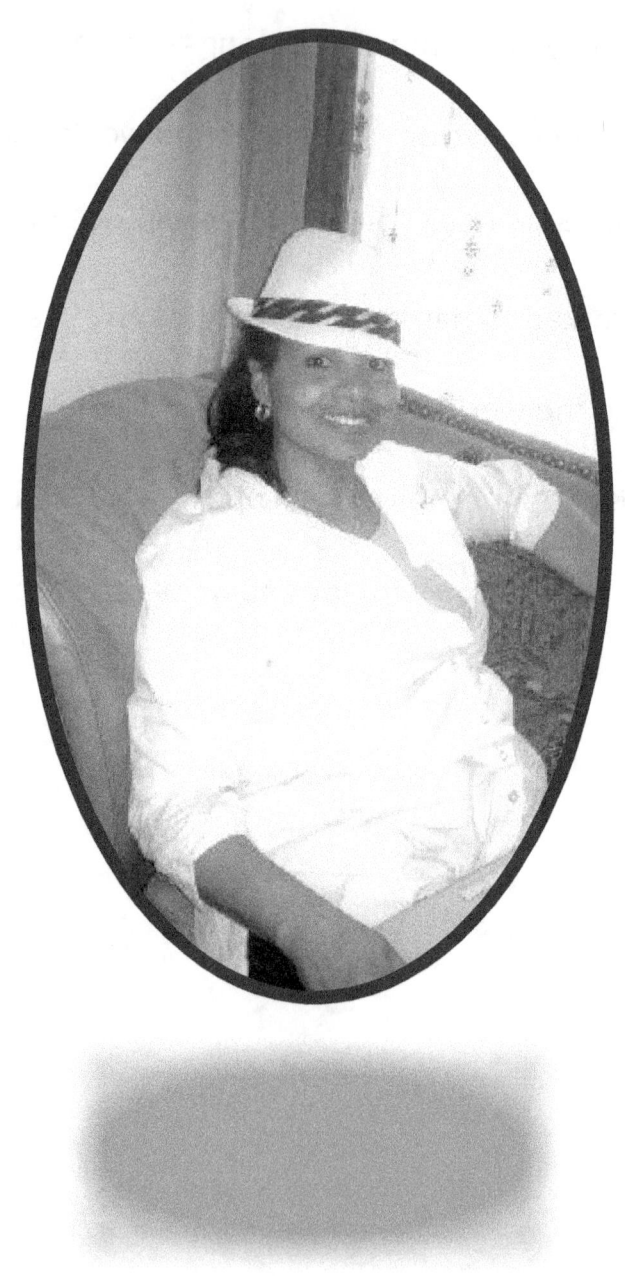

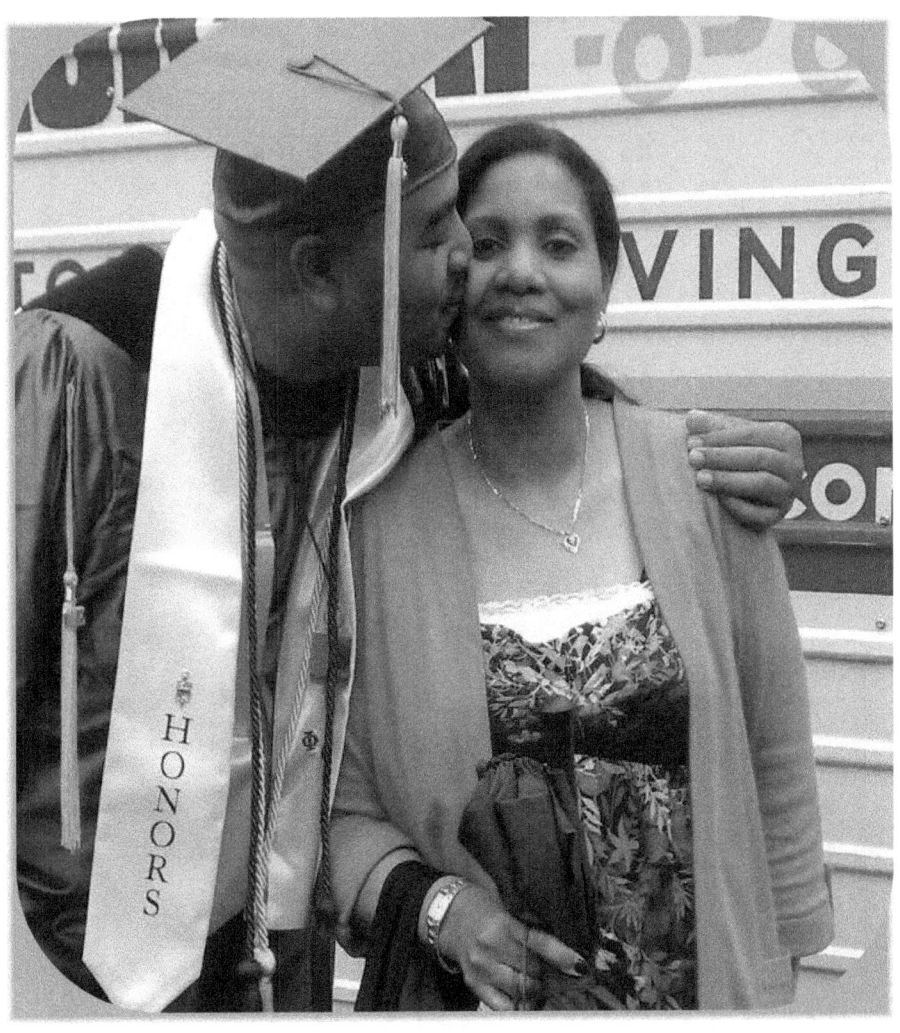

JOURNEY

INTO

LUPUS

"YVONNE

LIGHTNER'S STORY"

Authored By Gregory T. Lightner Jr

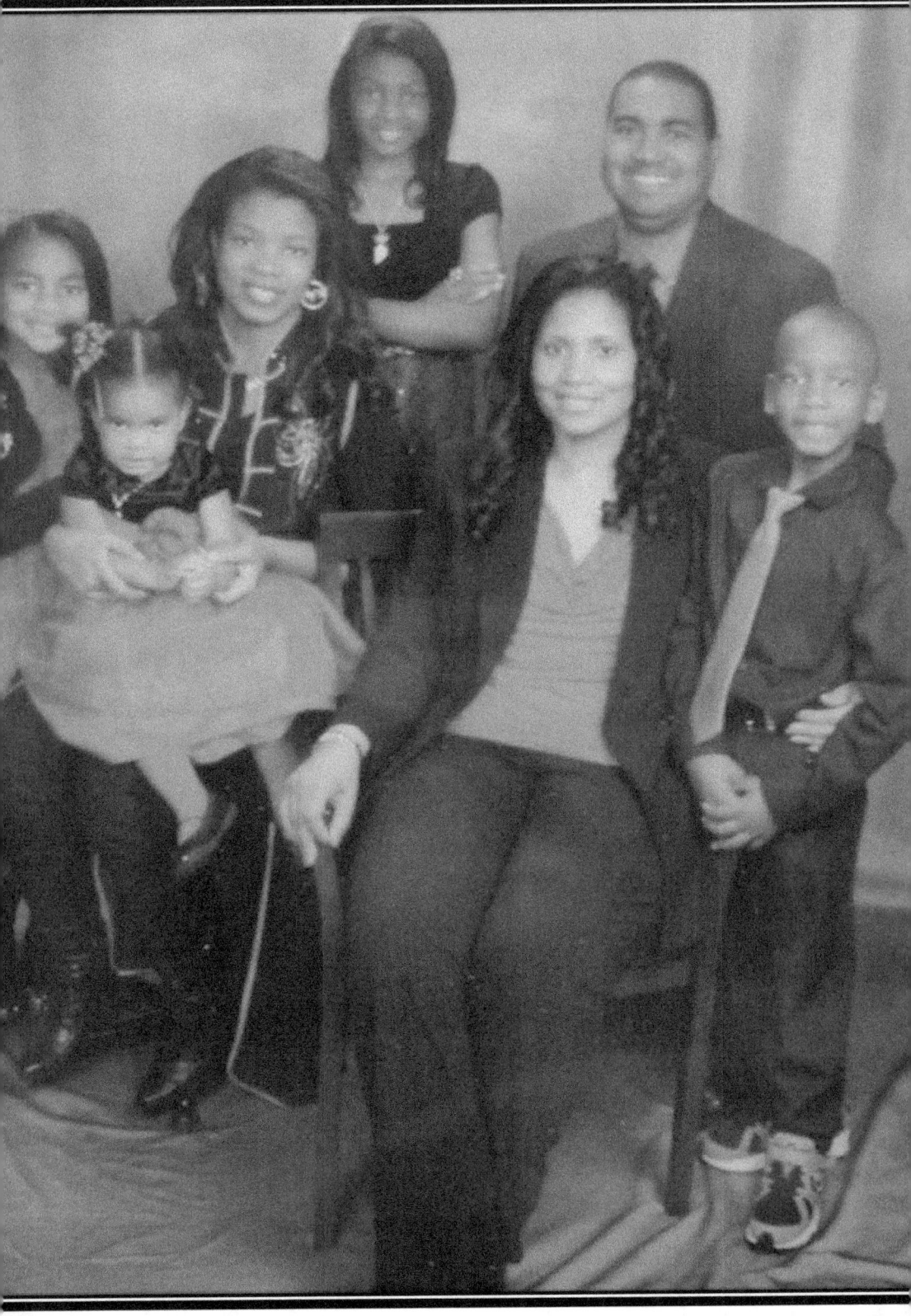

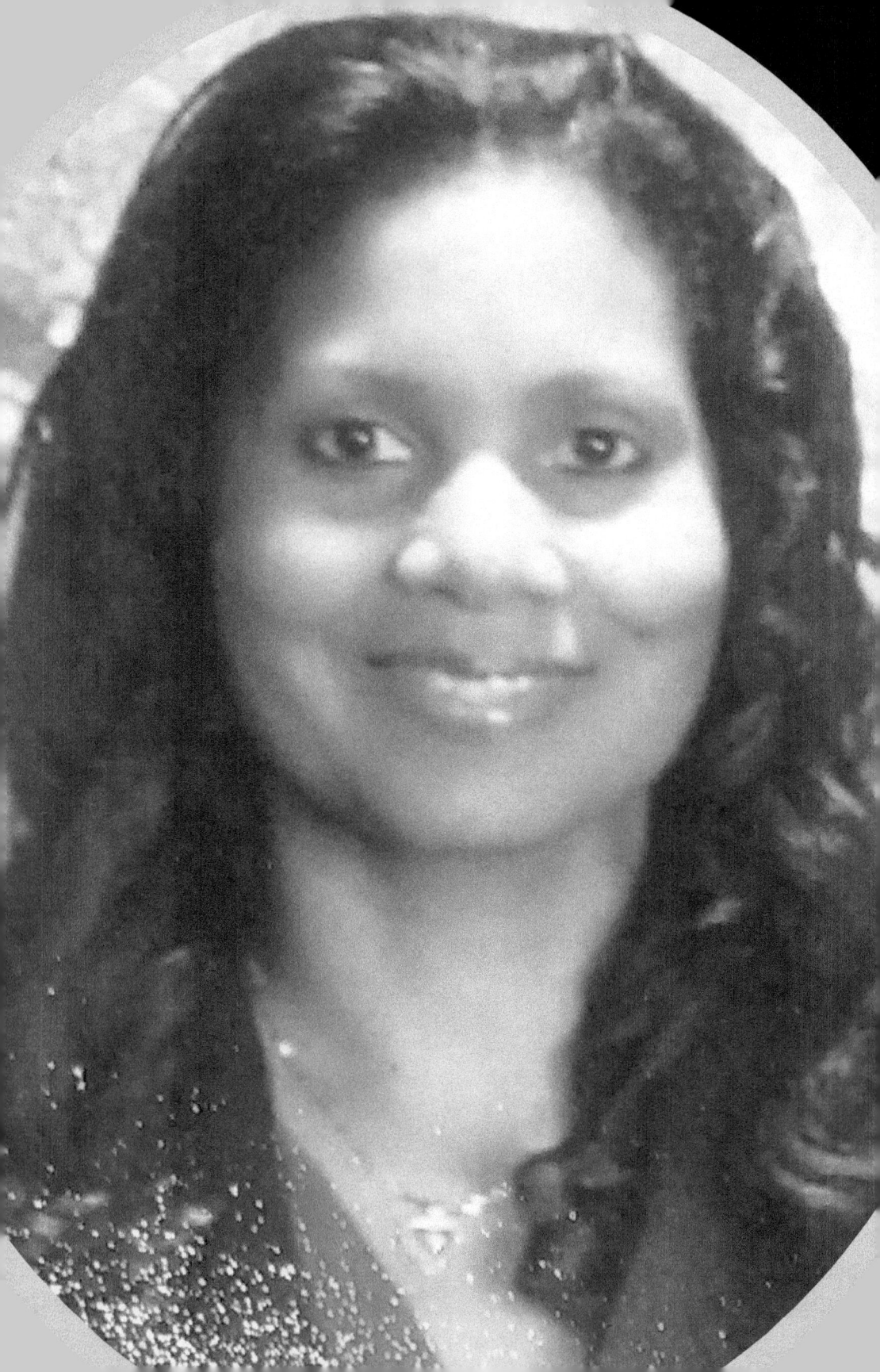

FROM THIS POINT ON YOU WILL HEAR THE VOICE OF YVONNE "IN HER OWN VOICE AND WORDS" MAY YOU BE TOUCH AS HER WORDS ECHO FROM THE HALLS OF THE MOST HIGH TO US HERE ON EARTH....

PEACE & BLESSINGS BE UPON YOU AND YOUR FAMILY!!!

INTRODUCTION

What motivated me to write this book sprung from being diagnosed with Lupus. I began a search for information detailing medical and personal accounts of the disease. Only to find that not a lot was out there; much of which was written twenty five to thirty or more years ago by doctors and the like; giving primarily a medical perspective. My goal was to continue searching for personal stories from your average person diagnosed, which at the time would have helped me tremendously in knowing that I was not alone in this experience.

To my disappointment there weren't any. So, throughout my entire illness, I began telling myself that once I survived this ordeal; I would be writing a book detailing my personal account of what

the experience was like going through

and surviving lupus. Therefore, having

hopes that this will somehow help to

inspire all who are in the struggle to

continue with the fight to live.

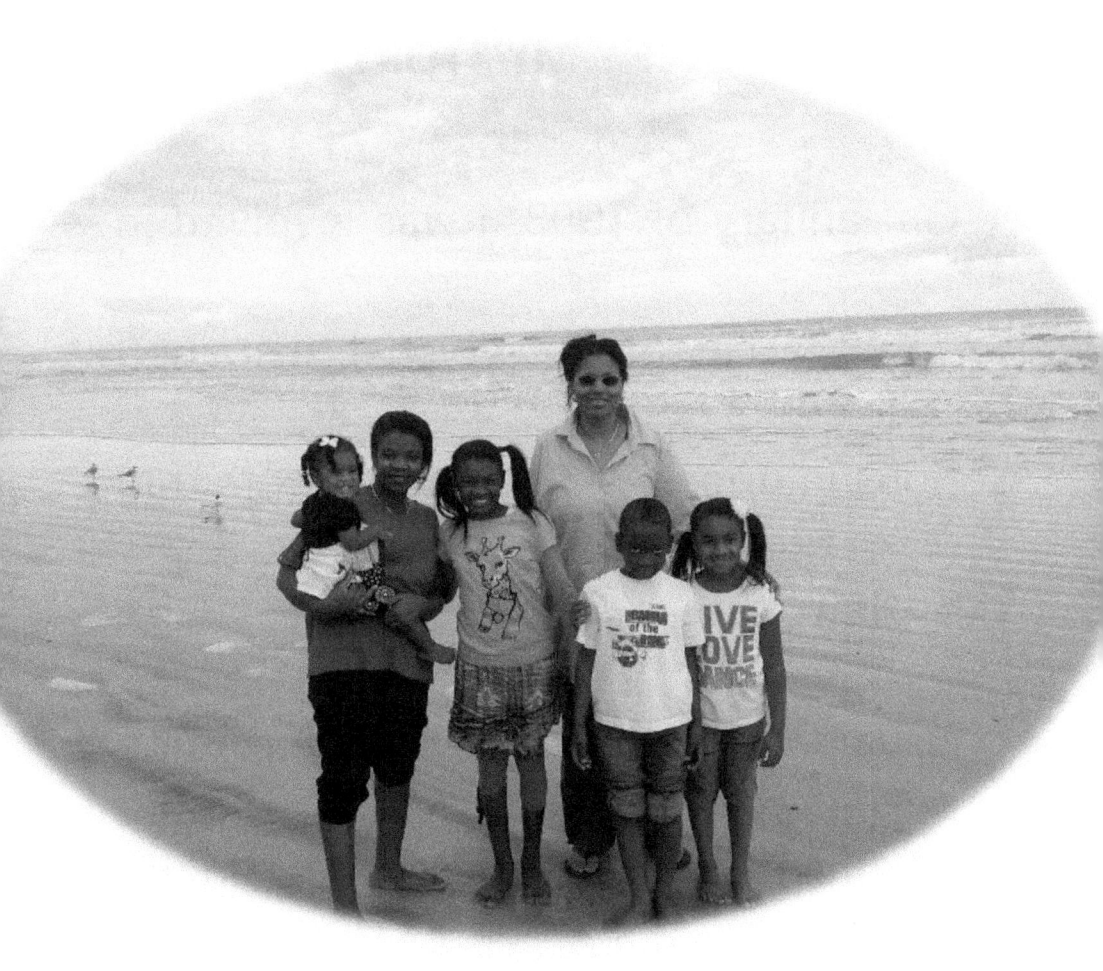

WHY MY STORY?

On January of 1993, I was involved in an auto accident, in which I sustained serious injuries. At first, the doctors told me that the symptoms were a bit unusual and to be considered routine and concurrent with the type of injury that I had sustained, but not to worry they were sure it was nothing serious. Little did I know, that the series of medical test that were to follow would

have such a profound impact on my life

and bring me face to face with the most

destructive and menacing demon called

LUPUS   [SLE]   Systemic   Lupus

Erythematosus.

INTROSPECTION

The expression "The earlier the better" is so often a part of our daily vocabulary, it has lost its ominous intention. As a Lupus survivor who has battled this disease, I implore all of you to be vigilant and remain proactive when it comes to lupus detection and recognition.

One of the greatest challenges you will face will be **Early** and **Correct** diagnosis, which is vital for maintaining your fragile health while reducing and even avoiding serious complications. I urge you to read this book in a setting that makes you most comfortable.

As we journey back into my life, it is my sincere hope that you may connect with me as if I am a friend or relative whom you can smile, cry and even laugh.

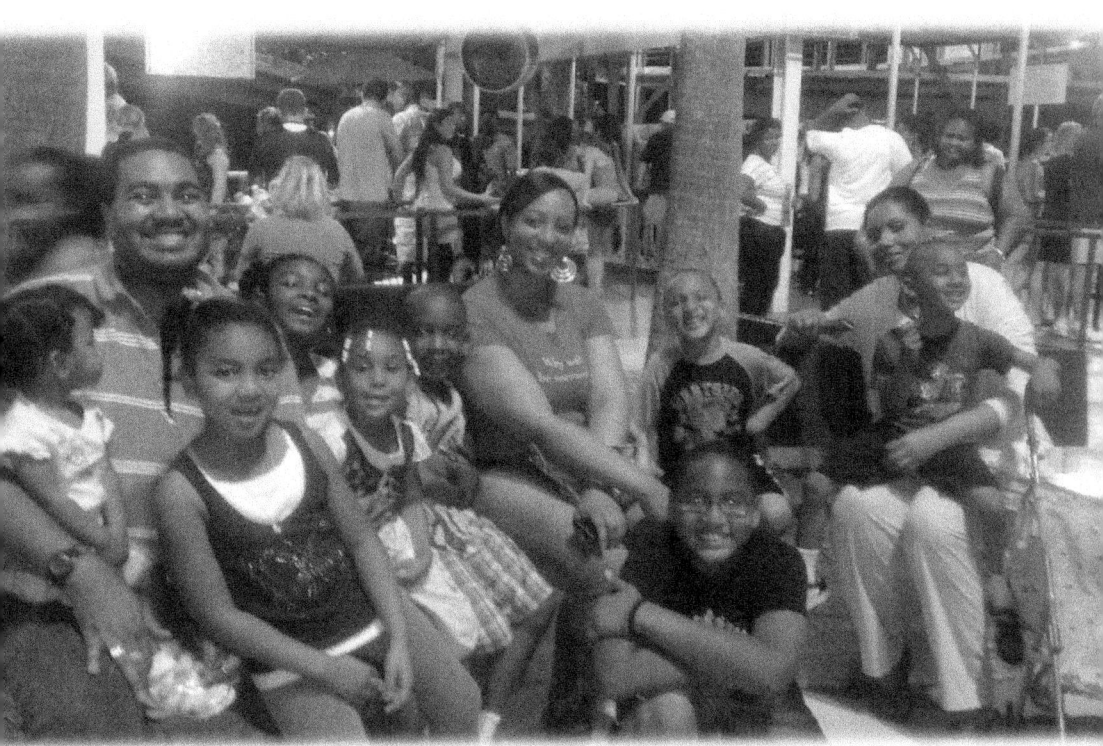

ECHOES OF THE PAST

The smells of fresh air, fruit fresh from the trees with a hint of lilac on a soft inviting breeze...

Reflections of my early childhood growing up on a small country farm, life was truly an enjoyable adventure. My loving siblings and I were always surrounded by a menagerie of animals and pets to interact and bond with.

One of the most vivid memories was of getting off of the school bus daily and being greeted by our pet geese. They would personally escorted us from the bus steps to our doorstep; was most delightful and also intriguing. Flush with excitement we would skip and run almost simultaneously, straight into our house to be mesmerized by the sweet aroma of cookies and muffins baking in the oven.

Hug & kisses were always in abundance as mom pleasantly welcomed us. As children we had very disciplined parents and fell into our daily routine quite efficiently. We would get changed as quickly as possible into our play attire, enjoy the delicious homemade snacks and complete our homework. It was only then that we were allowed to watch the "The Big Show" which was a very popular science fiction television program that we, would not dare to miss watching with mom. Often after the show ended, we'd go outdoors to play on the farm.

From the time we could crawl, were a very competitive family. Very driven, we would constantly challenge ourselves and each other to be the best. This was especially enjoyable as we competing with one another from sports to academics. Our parents were persistent and consistent in maintaining structure, discipline and order in the household. What made life enjoyable was that they balanced structural discipline with a healthy dose of quality family time. I can recall so clearly having discussions about the day's current events, while we also laughed, joked around and watched family TV programs together with the whole family. These were things provided to us to help in insuring that we all stayed informed, active and grounded, which was instrumental in our development. Life on a farm included having several large gardens and chores. To maintain this daily was not always easy. Nevertheless, in spite of all the work to be done, we managed for the most part to turn it into a fun venture with the skills we had been given and there was without a doubt never a dull moment.

Our summers often consisted of nature walks, swimming, bicycling, building and racing go carts. We always were having competitions of just about every sport associated with a ball. We had it all including horseback riding too. Our yard was always filled with children who came from all around the neighborhood just to participate.

Now it makes sense as I realize that there were times when I would struggle to keep up with everyone while playing outdoors, engaging in tumbling exercises, sprinting, cartwheels and many other activities. Many times as the sun began to set I would start to get severe inflammation in my throat, which would bring an abrupt end to playtime for me.

I would have to go indoors as everyone else continued on, leaving me feeling quite unhappy and disappointed. Many times these bouts of illness were accompanied by severe persistent aches and pains throughout my entire body, along with chronic swollen sore throat. Also I was plagued by chest and hip pain which began to affect every aspect of my young life.

One of the most devastating memories was the terrible reaction I suffered after getting an immunization (small pox vaccine). At the tender age of six that caused me to become extremely ill which in retrospect was a glimpse of things to come. Consequently, this was a life altering experience which I would not fully recover from.

In time, as difficult as it was I grew to accept my limitations and even at this tender young age my determination to defy all obstacles was starting to blossom .

Looking back as a teenager, if I had the chance to go back and counsel myself, I would have done things rather differently. As teenagers we feel invincible and neglect keeping appointments for routine doctor visits.

We may try to "work thru" what we may perceive as small annoying illnesses which always somehow manage to get out of our control. I can readily admit that I was no different as most teenagers in this regard. My wiliness to ignore many quantifiers was compounded by the fact that despite my early health related setbacks, I was quite active and participated in more activities than most teens my age. Basketball, baseball, tennis, and many academic clubs were among so of the favorites. Most importantly, participating in the honor society was most special to me. I was voted most likely to succeed, and had the privilege of playing in the honors marching band as an accomplished flautist. This was when my love for music flourished as I opened my mind and attain an eclectic taste in music from classical to pop. As such, this liberating experience allowed me to immerse myself to infuse the power of music into my very essence. Music for me had far reaching therapeutic inner workings as complex as a toccata.

During one of the many rehearsals I specifically recall an event during practice that again was my body indicating that a severe situation was at hand. During two long hours in the hot exhausting sun, I felt what I thought to be the sting of a spider piercing my skin.

This was the natural assumption I came

to after believing I may have walked

through a web. Immediately, I started to

experience pain in my throat.

Accompanied by an almost

simultaneous migraine headache, I

began to experience extreme nausea.

Additionally, a rash covering half of my

back that contained painful welts had

developed. Some of my band mate's

contacted the band director whom after

being made aware of the circumstances,

dismissed me from practice and urged

me to seek medical attention

immediately. My mom would later take

me to the doctor, during the visit I was

diagnosed and treated for hives,

tonsillitis and arthritis. I would go on to

have numerous bouts of the same. I can

determine that this was the beginning

stages of a disease that scientifically,

almost nothing was known about at the time. Otherwise, I managed to have a fairly normal adolescence while also working a part time job.

After graduating high school a year early, I made a decision to work full time. Temporarily delaying my dreams and aspirations of attending college right away. Ironically, making this decision would be a curse and a blessing in disguise. I began working long hours as I was very driven but it soon began to take a toll on me physically.

I began leaving and missing work quite often due to severe symptoms that included painful eczema, P.M.S., nosebleeds and headaches. As a result I was compelled to visit a Dermatologist and an ENT Specialist (ear, nose and throat specialist) the latter advised me to quit my job. He further went on to explain that with my immune system being severely compromised, I'd be better off seeking an occupation where that I would have absolutely no contact with the public. Basically, setting the scene for what was to come.

As I was considering taking his advice, my situation changed with a chance encounter that led to me meeting my husband to be.

He was someone who I thought was intelligent, caring, thoughtful, witty, dashingly handsome, charismatic, and charming. Most of the qualities I had hoped for in a soulmate. This combination made for great times, happy times in the beginning of our relationship.

Just prior to my twentieth birthday, we married and conceived our first born child (Gregory Jr.). Early on during the pregnancy, I was diagnosed with toxemia which forcing me to leave my job. This began a series of medical complications for the next two pregnancies and years to follow; creating a most stressful environment that would tests the most sacred vows of our marriage. My once stoic and seemingly unflappable husband began having difficulty in dealing with the stresses of daily life.

It was difficult for him to open up about what he was going through and as many people do, he would turn to alcohol and later substance abuse as a means of coping. I continued to watch a once happy and excellent husband and father slip further away. To the outside world he was a picture of perfection but at home behind that façade lay a man who was broken and severely stressed. He would often explode at home which of course was very poor judgment on his part. This would continue to escalate into physical and mental abuses; and began to wear away at the very fabric and structure of our relationship. Somehow we managed to see it through by taking it one day at a time. In so doing, we decided to stay the course, and had the great fortune of being blessed in the following years with two more bundles of joy; Solomon and later on Aaron, making the future of having a family definitely worth fighting for.

At times, I looked and felt the picture of health while raising our children; living what I thought to be to some extent an uncharacteristic life. By this time, having gone through several miscarriages early on that were unknowingly, a direct result of the Lupus that was hiding and developing inside of my body; my life was definitely not going quite as planned.

Specialist later informed me that because of major complications during each pregnancy, I may not be able to have more children; and was lucky to have successfully conceived the three that I had. Upon being given this information, I immediately experienced an epiphany which allowed me to see how very bless and fortunate I was.

In late April of 1981, I noticed what appeared to be scratches all over my upper torso Befuddled, I thought that perhaps I or my husband accidentally scratched me during the night while asleep. I didn't give it another thought as it seemed random. I wish I had paid more attention to that detail because a few years later while interacting in activities & playing sports with my children (football, basketball, baseball, kickball), I began to bruise and tire easily, at times nearly passing out. My boys started to question why I no longer wanted to participate in their daily sports of little league baseball, basketball and football. In fact, the truth was that I did not have the strength, or the energy to keep up with them any longer.

Not wanting to cause additional fears and anxieties in my children, I continued to play down the fact that I may becoming seriously ill. My fears were confirmed subsequently when the phantom scratches reappeared. This time they were accompanied with rashes, fatigue, nosebleeds, and extreme bouts of dizziness and bruises that covered my entire body. It seemed that I could no longer hide even from my own fears. I became alarmed enough to seek medical attention, and was advised by my primary care doctor, *"You need not to worry, the rash is due to eczema."* As is customary, prescriptions were taken and the rash along with everything else disappeared, "The end"—so I thought. I began to work outdoors quite often gardening as way to relax. I was very passionate about it and it was just what I needed, to escape from the constant administrative demands of running our incredibly demanding plumbing contracting business. It was this very activity that led the realization sun sensitivity was becoming a major issue. Consequently, I had to almost completely curtail my outdoor activities. My health continued to deteriorate and simultaneously my ability to be the consummate jack of all trades was beginning to wane.

Eventually, I was forced to give up participating in the day to day duties of operating the family business due to my extensive medical problems.

March of 1993 was the first time I had even heard the term Lupus. After a routine thyroid exam and an extensive diagnostic tests; I was diagnosed with Lupus (SLE) and ITP- (idiopathic thrombocytopenic purpura) an autoimmune and bleeding disorder associated with low platelets. The levity of condition did not set in until after having a traumatically, terrifying and extremely painful bone marrow extraction. Shortly after arriving home from the procedure my phone rang... It was a frantic call from my doctor who seemed a bit unnerved, stated in a quivering yet authoritative tone voice, "Go back to the hospital immediately!

No time to explain, I will meet you there...." My husband had pick up the other phone and was at a loss for words. When he came in to our bedroom I was still standing with the phone in my hand. He came over and gently took the phone from my hand and said ever so softly, "Pooh Bear, we will get through this...I promise." In that moment the man whom I admired so much was again standing, ready to take on the world.

Our children walked in and we all embraced with a moment of eerie silence that I wish would never be broken. This was a stark blow that stated unequivocally my condition had become progressively worse. After arrive at the hospital I was told that my platelets were dangerously low so much that I was in desperate need of transfusion (gamma globulin).In the subsequent discussion with my husband

I was concerned of the implications and more disconcerting, the dangers. My husband was able to quell my fears and begrudgingly I agreed. The transfusion was successful for the time being but nothing lasts forever, I would then go on to have several more transfusions and a subsequent hospital stay October, 1993 before it was all over.

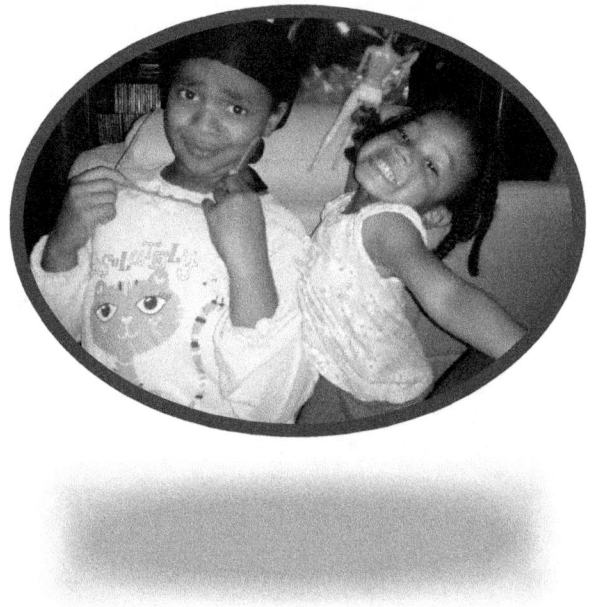

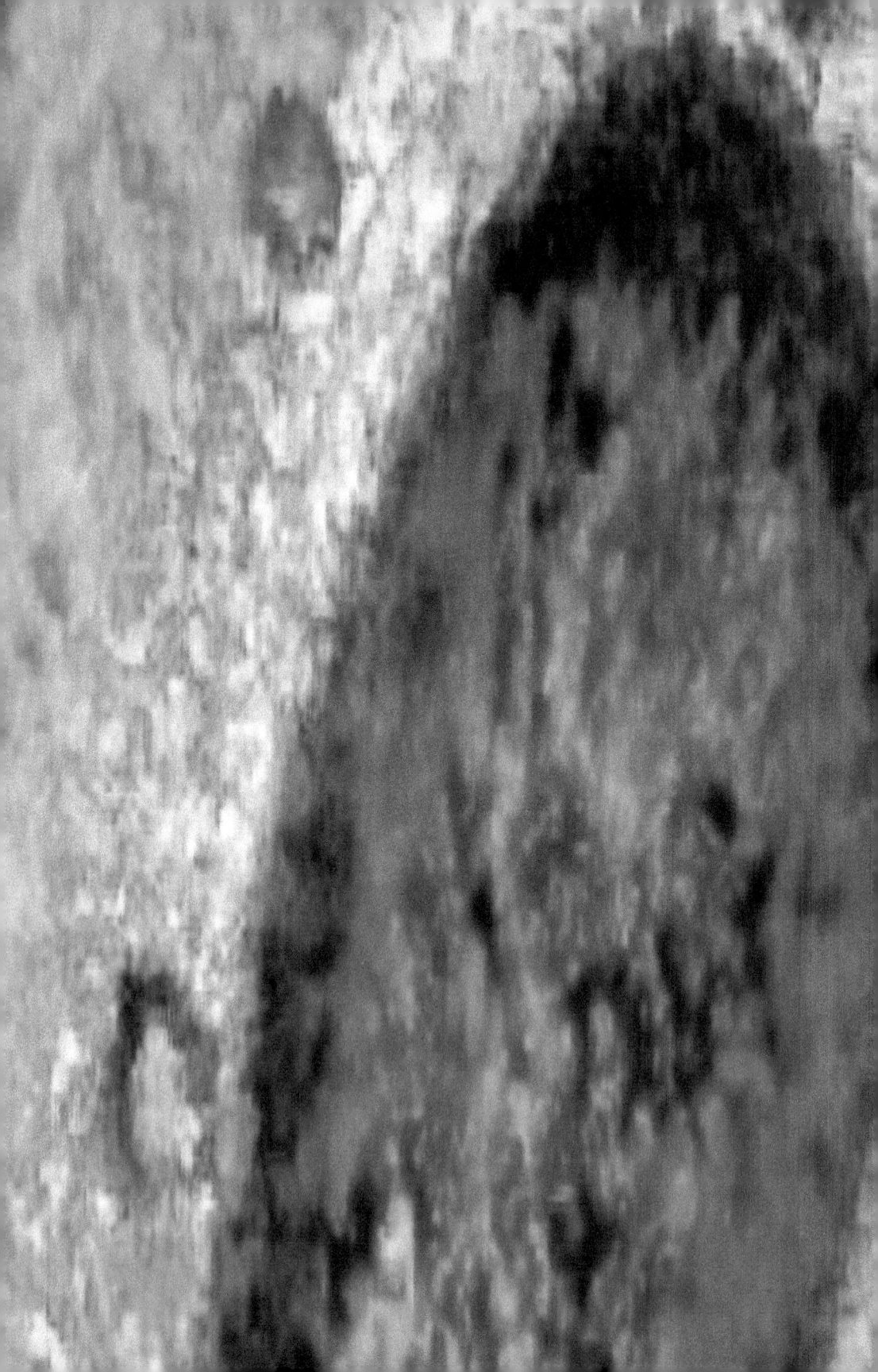

FREEFALL INTO THE ABYSS

Meanwhile, the maze of madness; tunnel of darkness and uncertainty had just begun, leaving me at times feeling totally lost, confused, disillusioned and helpless. Though, thru it all, I began to think in terms of fighting this thing, this demon of destruction. A monster of unimaginable cruelty and wickedness.

There was not a **snowballs chance in hell** I would allow it to control me. I was defiantly determined not to give up or in, I would continue on like a battle weary warrior that was condemned to run a gauntlet. This was the moment of reckoning, an uphill battle for my life.

Life went on difficult challenges but forward none the less. I enjoyed a vibrant social life and was quite content until the dreaded "D" word declared war on my mind. Dementia began to creep upon me and settle in. It was a thief in the night, with no mercy attacking my mind constantly. All the while, my body was continuing to ache constantly. Lupus was waging a steady methodical war which was relegating me with each passing day to a monotonously dreadful enslavement ripe with pain and confusion.

I spent so much time lying down that I came to refer to my bed as, "The miserable bed of nails." I looked upon it as a tormentor, trickster, menacing curse, determined to slowly draining the life out of me. The mere thought of dusk, brought on a feeling of total doom and dread coupled with anxiety. My body would always respond to the changes in atmosphere, solar events, and lunar patterns such as the rise and fall of the sun the moon. It was hard to fathom something like that causing such excruciating pain and discomfort that most times, I could barely sleep throughout the night or during the day. Unfortunately, sleep was not a source of comfort or relaxation for me.

Many times, I would awake to excruciating joint and muscle pain; so severe that I could not lift myself up out of bed, or even open my mouth to speak for at least an hour or more (manifestation of TMJ). Breakfast consisted of only liquids administered through a straw. At which time, I'd have to literally pry open my mouth with just enough space to insert a straw. I would then have to get assistance from family members; taking away what I considered to be the last of my independence, which made me even more determined to fight this demon of darkness.

A simple touch became similar to what can be described as the sensation of shards of glass being thrust underneath my skin. Every day the approaching afternoon meant, severe joint/muscle pain, and stiffness combined with debilitating headaches. Most of the times the suffering would end up rendering me completely motionless, helpless, and at times virtually paralyzed. At times I was reduced to eye movement as the only means of communication. The only salvation and refuge I had to get me through the nights were my prayers. Sometimes in my darkest moments I'd pray for death to overtake me. But somehow I willed myself away from the despair and returned to positive thoughts. The most defiant was always *"You are not going to win—I will conquer you!!!(Lupus)."* It became a ritual of sorts, most days and nights were spent repeating these words. This phrase would be repeated many times over for the next several months and years; all the while I was holding onto this small bit of belief in myself and I was in control of my destiny, not the Lupus.

Soon it became increasingly difficult to converse with others anyone leaving me to feel even more isolated and disconnected from the world. No longer having the ability to articulate my thoughts and feelings made it all the more troublesome, being that our household was so full of scintillating conversation. I began to find myself withdrawing from the very things I had considered most important in life (family and friends). In fact, this was a defense mechanism used to protect myself, as well as, others from the pain and anguish that I endured. Reasoning became quite irrational. I no longer felt loved or needed. I had begun to feel as though my parents were my only hope of survival; all the while being within arm's reach of what I needed; my children. My thoughts were to run—run as far away as possible to Mom, Dad and my siblings where I'd surely find love, peace, comfort and understanding. So I waited until the summer to come and as soon as my children were out of school for summer break I packed up and left for two months. What I was seeking in my parents and siblings I did find for a short time. This was a time of reflection that allowed me to remember who I was, where I was and where my life was going. Ultimately this snapping me back into reality, I had gained momentary clarity which felt good—if only for a short time.

After returning to my life back home I was faced with tremendous problems, and all rational began to fade. The downward spiral into darkness had begun again as I became increasingly agitated due to the agony of severe sleep deprivation. It was a dreadful cycle would allow one to three hours of continuous sleep on a good night. My mind was always racing, voraciously consumed with erratic waves of uncontrollable thought, never to rest. The irritation was unbearable as the simplest of things would irritate me greatly. My unease was further exasperated and began to manifest as extreme paranoia, which magnified the most negative aspects of my marriage which, resulted in a most unfavorable relationship with my husband and children.

There are events that I recall as pivotal memories. In particular, there was one time shortly after my return home when I withstanding an unrelenting barrage of verbal attacks from my husband who proceeded uninhibited. I snapped and made a decision to make life for him as miserable and uncomfortable as possible.

I found it impossible to not dwell on every single transgression related and otherwise to our relationship. My mission each day was to make him as miserable as he had made me over the years. Not realizing that I'd only be hastening the effects of the disease, I was harming my own psyche with this unnecessary stress. Clearly, this was irrational and yet another phase of the dark progression and manifestations of dementia in the works.

No matter how bleak the results were the love of my children always prevailed. Most often, their infectious laughter, quick wit, and sense of humor would somehow pull me back from the darkness. They made it possible for me to laugh from time to time during this altered state. Often when coming home they never grew weary of telling countless jokes to lighten the mood always lifting my spirits.

Another enduring memory is of my son Aaron. In he strolled to the house and came into my bedroom, while I happened to be sitting in bed deeply depressed, angry and sulking. He began making gestures pointing to his face, then to mine jokingly uttering, *"Apple pie..., apple pie...!"* referring to the shape of my face due to bloating. This would always cause me to break out in hysterical laughter, just as I had lost all hope of ever living a normal existence; making me realize that all was not as bad as it seemed.

I thank my heavenly father for granting my children the ability to persevere in the face of despair; by means of using humor when faced with the unthinkable.

DIVINE INTERVENTION

By September of 1996, the over-whelming stresses of daily life dealing with three very active teenage boys combined with the demands of motherhood, an abusive (physically & verbally) dysfunctional, volatile marital relationship which lacked any moral support or means of constructive communication, life became far too much for me to bear. For instance, one day while out grocery shopping, my legs and feet began to feel as if I were dragging lead weights around and I barely managed to get back to my vehicle. By the time I arrived back home, my body was covered in bruises and hemorrhages from head to toe. This was a result of stress combined with and an unknown allergic reaction after consuming too many mango fruit; causing my condition to become critical. Realizing that time was of the essence, I attempted to contact my doctor but was in such a weakened state mentally and physically, that I could hardly summon up the strength to speak. This would, result in an immediate prolonged hospital stay September 25, 1996. This event subsequently opened the second door into my journey through the nightmare of Lupus, filled with shattered fragments of memories and terrifying experiences.

It was such an awful experience that is difficult to fathom. While lying in my hospital bed being administered an intravenous transfusion of gamma globulin and having my platelets replaced, I literally felt my life slipping away and fought to hold on. Voices were calling out to me whispering, *"Yvonne...Yvonne...Yvonne!"* though I was alone in the room. This would be my initial encounter with one of many near death experiences. As I began to drift in and out of consciousness, a tunnel appeared before me. I was curious and wanted to see what this was with such a tiny bright white light in the distance. As I started to gravitate towards and into this tunnel I felt a floating sensation as I was swirling along similar to the inside of a kaleidoscope. Suddenly what I can best describe as a giant fog-like translucent hand appeared in front of me. It began pushing me back to the entrance of this tunnel, when the face of my father materialized behind this hand. Back in my hospital bed, I opened my eyes startled by what had just occurred when my senses became heightened. I heard and felt someone come into my room but it wasn't a nurse or doctor.

I glanced over to my left and moving towards me was this shadowy figure. I was frozen and confused as the form took shape, larger than life it was my deceased baby brother. He continued towards me eventually passing through me and the bed before evaporating into the wall. Stunned, I soon realized that a nurse had also entered the room about the same time to take my vitals. She simply smiled and said, *"Looks like someone has a guardian angel watching over her."* To which I whispered, *"Did you see that too?"* and she said, *"Yes (with a smile) he's a big guy, who was that?"* And I said, *"My baby brother."* She also commented that, *"You would not believe some of the things we've seen."*

Shortly thereafter, my condition improved enough for me to be released and I thought that all would be ok. The day I was back home and upon collecting my thoughts, I called my parents informing them about what I had witnessed and gone through. I remember asking, *"What do you think this means?"* my question was met with eerie, almost ominous silence. The period after my release, would be an incredibly short period of recovery

similar to the eye of a hurricane.

THE FINAL JOURNEY

On October 15, 1996, my third and

final hospital stay, which I'll call the final

journey; culminated into the most

frightening, and surreal experience of

my life. A journey, that took on a life of

its own as unexplainable, unbelievable

and miraculous occurrences. The

unpredictability of this condition makes the journey all the more perplexing. This here is my version unedited and unfiltered as accurately as I can recall.

On October 15th 1996 my day began at approximately 6:30 am after a sleepless night. I had a feeling of uneasiness that I could not shake as I sat listlessly on the side of my bed. I was waiting to be driven to the hospital for what I thought would be a five day stay of certainty. Strangely the phone rang shortly after 7:00 am literally just as I was about to leave. I knew it was horrible news by the look on my husband's face. It was a call informing me of my father's passing. I remember thinking, *"This can't be happening again, I'm still grieving the loss of Paul!"* (My youngest brother). Obviously this news added to my distressed already confused fragile state of mind—I had no choice; my priority was getting admitted immediately to the hospital for treatment, for I was in poor health. I headed for the hospital and upon being admitted medications were administered almost immediately. That first day I became confused, lethargic and agitated.

The following day was the beginning of a period of medical uncertainty. I was found by my nurse curled up in bed with a massively swollen head and neck. A Lupus flair up the likes of which I had never experience had begun completely delirious, forced to navigate the darkest recesses of my tormented mind. The sound of jacks being tossed and shaken; sounds escalating; jacks were morphing into a huge ball as high as the ceiling; sounds becoming unbearable to the extreme of covering my ears and screaming out; *"Stop, Stop! Please make it stop!!"* not knowing where I was drifting in and out of consciousness. Finally, it stopped!

During the time of being found unresponsive and curled up in a fetal position, there came a point when I was completely aware of conversations going on around me. A team of doctors (specialist) entered the room and began discussing and consulting with one another about my prognosis. I recall them standing at my bedside carrying on in conversation as if I were not even there. And shortly after their departure, my husband and children entered my room with doctors and nurses and began to argue about why my condition had deteriorated so drastically in such a short time. They began to question what types of medications were given. I specifically recall them asking, *"Did anyone give her aspirin?"* Which they denied, but I knew otherwise, and could not verbally communicate this at the time.

So as they continued to stand over me arguing back and forth demanding a more plausible explanation, apparently my youngest son Aaron had been at my side quietly sitting by the window watching over me. In this moment it was almost like I was able to telepathically reach out and connect with Aaron. He began to verbalize every thought process I had concerning what was occurring, which was miraculous. He essentially became my voice at this time eventually, telling them that a young male nurse had given me aspirin, as well as, making other mistakes. He further demanded that they immediately contact my primary care doctor for my medical history.

With the understanding that my family was there looking out for my safety; I slipped back into a total state of unconsciousness; only to awaken later to total madness that was almost incomprehensible. This leaves me to assume that this was the progression of me spiraling into a two week coma.

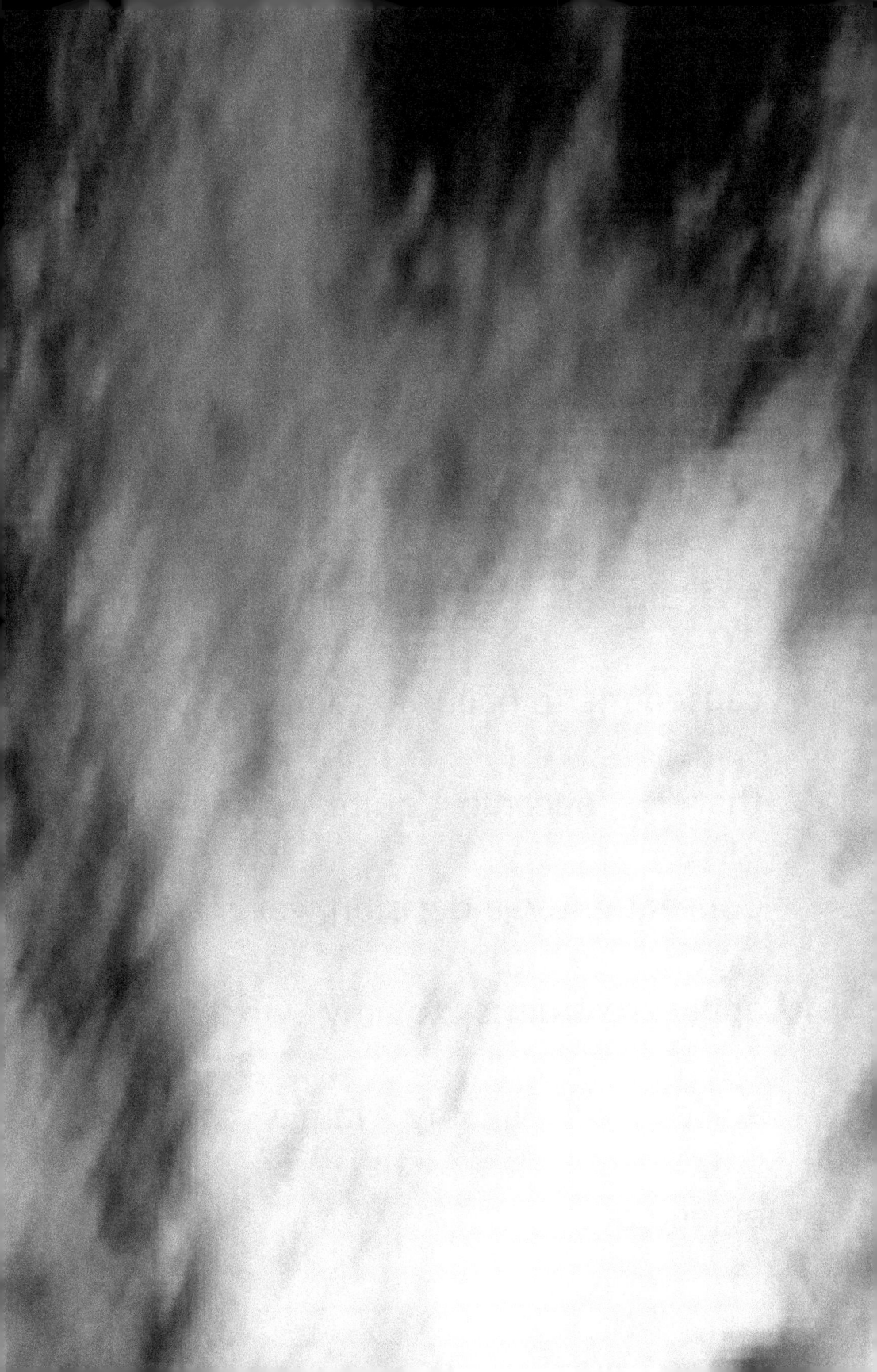

HALLUCINATIONS

With the development of massive swelling of my head and body; edema and allergic reactions to medications caused me to hallucinate to the extent that I became quite combative. Consequently, a decision was made to apply restraints to my wrists and ankles, which my family bitterly objected.

Their constant vigilance and bitter demands forced the removal of the restraints. Medications were again administered to quell and suppress the episodes and once the medication began to take effect, the hallucinations began to explode upon my mind with devastating detonation.

The best way to illustrate this seeming unreal experience is list each episode individually, along brief description of some of the bizarre and unimaginable hallucinations that I began to experience during this time. My hope is that if you have lupus or know someone who does my experience can help you understand just how tough it can be............

1. Being at my father's funeral; watching the service from the inside of his dark blue coffin; observing family and friends while mourning. The lid was closed; I began to claw and scream; awoke to sound of machine beeping, back in CCU.

2. My fathers' coffin being carried into hospital room, falling and crushing one of my brother's toes; could hear bones cracking.

3. Falling into a dark hole; an abyss with a net and making several attempts to jump out, as if I were on a trampoline, before finally propelling myself out; all appearing very animated.

4. Intruders who had breached security in hospital came in solely to attack me. One intruder managed to get through, came in with a gun and shot me six times through the heart while verbalizing expletives; then turns and escapes. Leaving me clutching my chest—I died.

5. Sliding in and out of reality (lying in hospital bed trying to make sense of what was currently happening and what was not).

6. Seeing myself as a corpse pronounced dead, placed in body bag and wheeled into the hospital morgue.

7. Fighting with hospital staff (punching, hitting) thinking they were trying to inflict bodily harm.

8. Visualizing an elderly woman of 80 whom was very selfish and cruel, who said *"no"* to everyone and everything while unable to walk, would drag and scoot heavy chair across floor making loud irritating dragging sounds to get to and from.

9. A small boy of eight, precocious and inquisitive questioning everything and everyone.

10. Seeing my brother attacking a nurse breaking her jaw, cursing, ranting raging. Then, being beaten up by hospital security, and eventually succumbing to his injuries.

11. Seeing how my mom, dad and two aunts died. (Currently all are deceased except for mom.)

12. Distortion of blood transfusion (clotting blood going into tubes).

13. Choking a female doctor for antagonizing me about my appearance saying, *"Your eyes are out to here! Do you want a mirror?"* and demonstrating.

14. Air bubbles moving through IV drip; tried to pull out.

15. Hot light bulb touching and burning my left arm whenever I reached over to rip out IV tubing.

16. An elderly gentleman found dead inside of my room. Orderlies came in to remove his body. The corpse continued moaning and groaning while being abused by them; breaking bones as they prepared to place him inside of a body bag.

17. Lying in bed defenseless while seeing a dusting of multicolored particles of light sprinkled above my head; feeling enormous pressure in head and eyes. The top of my head exploding: **Poof!!**—like a powder puff; causing me to flinch. At which point, I could see doctors and nurses peering down inside of my head, while the head nurse began shouting mean and disgusting things to me about myself and family.

Amazingly, my eyes appeared to view this all from the top of my brain. I then watched myself awaken from coma.

After about two weeks (according to medical records) just as I thought it was all over, another frightening door opened.   Regaining   consciousness thereafter, I questioned why so many clergy of all faiths/denominations were visiting my room. A *Doctor responded;* *"Your husband gave permission, and don't quote me on this, but it resembled a scene out of the exorcist."*

I do believe this to be absolutely true from the terror/fear etched on each and everyone's face upon entering my room; as all appeared to be moving about in slow motion. Since that time, I have begun recalling snippets of details surrounding this period such as; uncontrolled back and forth turning of my head, growling, ranting, raging, cursing and lashing out at everyone. Then becoming extremely annoyed at the procession of clergy as they scurried about carrying incense and reciting prayers along with quoting scriptures. At the same time, an oppressive feeling of malevolence continues to engulf me; making me feel as though I were a minuscule object, and that the true me were shrinking; being devoured by some demonic force trying to take over and control me.

But refusing to surrender, I began silently calling out asking for God to help me; *"Please heavenly father, help me!"*

with great trepidation as I recited the lords' prayer……. God heard my cry; lifting the veil of darkness.

This also brings to mind what occurred weeks later during a post hospital visit. I asked one of my doctors why he and others appeared to have age over night; he responded, pointing to his almost completely grey hair, *"You did this to me, don't ask and do not try to remember; you would not want to know...."* [And I thank you heavenly father for pulling me back; rescuing me from the brink of insanity and darkness].

Incidentally, later someone remarked that pictures should have been taken of me during this time, because otherwise no one will ever believe what they had all witnessed. However, out of curiosity, I continued to press my husband and children for more information

surrounding this period, and found that

the subject was not something they

cared to give further details about.

Obviously, the memory of this situation

was too horrific and disturbing to even

want to recall. The subject was not

brought up again until years later only to

be met with the same unwillingness, and

was further told that they would never

speak of it again. After that, my decision

was to just let it be; it was not that important.

With that being said, given such unusual circumstances I can only surmise that this experience had a profound affect; some negative, some positive on all who were involved with my case.

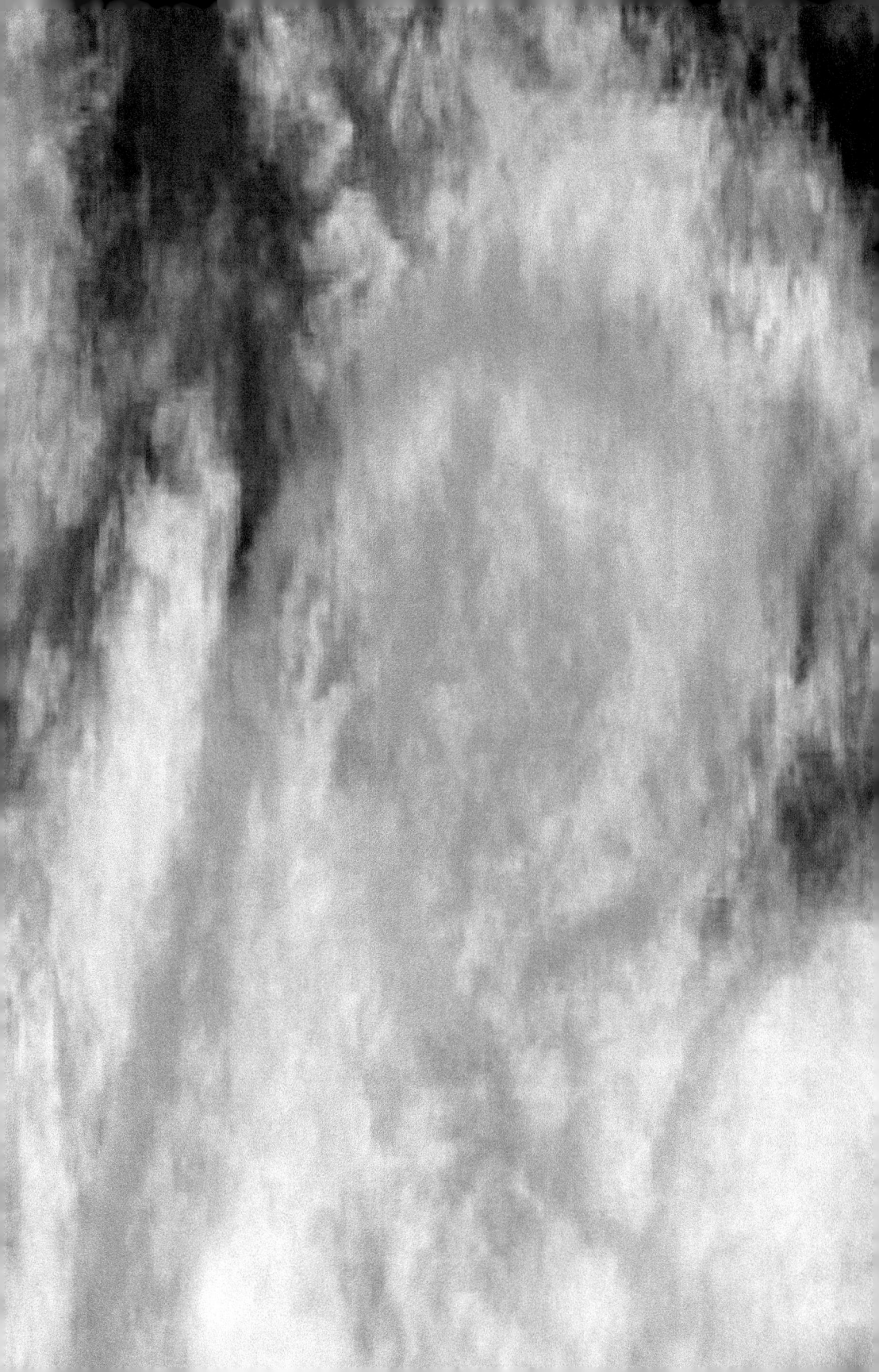

A FATHER HELPS FROM BEYOND

While restless and disoriented I

watched as my deceased father

entered my room. The room began

to fill with the most spectacular

flowers of beauty, and with each

step, unfolding more flowers (roses

and flowers of all kinds) along with

an abundance of love and peace

that washed over me. He sat down at my bedside; beside me. Placing his hand on my knee reassuringly saying, *"Yvonne honey, everything is going to be just fine, "Daddy loves you; now rest"* and I did. Daddy came to my rescue from beyond, just as he promised he would during my last visit home prior to his passing; apparently, this too took place during the time my head and neck were swollen due to an allergic reaction to medication (Rocephin) that was given, and was never given again. I was later told that my head had swollen to almost the size of a standard size bed pillow, and that my eyeballs were protruding beyond the eye sockets, whereas enabling visually to see behind the eyes *[diagnosed as severe case of conjunctivitis]*.

My doctor would later visit my room and ask me if I knew where my father was—I assume this may also have been his way of testing the scope of my cognitive abilities—I responded, *"Yes, he's dead..."* Doctor appeared to be baffled. He then turned and walked away, leaving specific orders with the attending nurses to continue closely monitoring me.

As a result, I became agitated with the nurse sitting at the foot of my bed staring— what I perceived at the time as rudely staring. My understanding of her reason for being there observing me was not registering. I was unaware of my condition and appearance, and did not react kindly to her stares. After saying and doing God knows what to the poor woman, she got up with a look of complete fright and

tearfully exited quickly.

Looking back on this incident had

the roles been reversed, as a

professional I am sure I would have

reacted in the same manner as the

nurse. However, I was unapologetic

and quite relieved to see her no

longer caring for me.

Afterwards, staff members placed a call to my husband Gregory Sr. requesting that he return to the hospital immediately to help in calming me down. Shortly thereafter, he came in, sat down next to my bed, and began admonishing me about my behavior; telling me to calm down and be quiet saying, *"I'll be right here, now stop antagonizing the nurses for doing their job, doing*

what they were told to do."

Reluctantly, I did as he asked of

me; relaxing and falling back

asleep. That night he slept in a

chair beside my bed. A staff

member told me later on that my

husband and children were the

only ones to have a calming effect

on me during these episodes

which proved to be very helpful to

all involved.

COMA

While on a respirator, sounds of machines pumping irritated me. I felt intense pressure building inside of my head and eyes. I began to panic as I visualized my eyes and brain bleeding, blood vessels in both gorged with blood; gradually swelling and protruding in a continuous progression; just prior to exploding while I continued without a sound to beg and plead for God's help.

Then just as my eyes erupted like a volcano, everything stopped abruptly! Voices called out from shadowy figures whom I believed to be guardian angels suspended above my body saying, ***"rollback! rollback!"*** sending everything swiftly into reverse mode; rewinding and revealing every single detail of the swelling as it took place from start to finish, but in this instance from finish to start. I began seeing my body lying suspended in air; over red-hot coils in a hospital room slowly rotating; like a rotisserie for what seemed like hours to several days. Heat radiated up and down my body from head to toe slowly inching along; healing as it continued to rotate. Heat was not as we know it to be here on earth; was only inches away; skin did not burn; only the disease inside was gradually being destroyed and forever eradicated.

Upon awakening after two weeks of lying in a comatose state, a nurse standing at my bedside shouted out, *"she's back, she's back, get a doctor in here!"* as I attempted to play possum, but my vitals gave me away. She asked

me to open my eyes saying, *"We know*

that you can hear us, now can you open

your right hand and move your fingers—

can you wiggle your toes for us... blink

once for yes and two for no..." Slowly

opening my eyes, I struggled to do as

instructed but could only move my left

less dominant side. In addition, I was so

extremely weak and could not speak, sit

unassisted, stand or walk. Lying in bed

completely immobilized and frozen with

fear, the realization of complete nursing

staff dependence set in. Nurses were

coming and going as I tried to

communicate; (verbally and in writing)

my complaints of discomfort from an

agonizing bed sore and heel pain. At the

time, I felt as if air became a substitute

for my brain; my mind went completely

blank as my thoughts faded quickly. By

the time I rang my call bell the thoughts

were gone. The nurses would respond as I struggled to remember why I called for assistance; leaving me to apologize for my lapses in memory. These episodes continued to occur numerous times over a period of days to weeks.

Meanwhile, in cases where patients are diagnosed as being in a comatose state; be very careful of the conversations you have in their presence. My reason for saying this is that, when I was in this state, there were many private/personal conversations and comments going on between personnel in front of me; assuming that I was unaware of what was being said. But, I heard all, some of what was quite disturbing. Although, I certainly understand how demanding the job can be; patients should not be subjected to personal bickering amongst staff members, or anyone for that matter. In situations such as this; try to be more mindful of the human being lying there stuck in between two worlds.

Then there came the time of being reintroduced to eating. It was thought by nurses that I was being stubborn and difficult when I adamantly refused to eat. However, in actuality I was having difficulty with holding my utensils using my left hand instead of my right hand. A nurse helping me asked, *" Aren't you right handed... so why are you using your left hand for everything...?"* leaving me to ponder...

As I attempted to eat, swallowing became very difficult. My throat would start to close whenever I'd try to drink or eat a little bit. With every mouthful came a feeling of choking.

Eventually, my son Gregory realized what was happening, and made an decision to be present for and take charge to proceed slowly and with caution concerning my feedings (food and drink consumption). I still don't know how he was able to make such a sacrifice that would change his life for good. My first born dropped everything to be here for his mom.

There would also be a time, when waking up, that my muscles began to atrophy. I began screaming and shrieking out from shin and leg pain, warranting an immediate course of pump circulation stimuli applied to my legs. My entire body became wracked with pain, so much so, that I mentally shut down to block out all of the pain and was given a sedative, as well. My organs began to shut down; going into total organ failure. I awoke again to see a grossly, massively distended abdomen, and a nurse standing before me pleasantly asking, *"Can you please try to urinate for me, and may I help you wash your hair once you feel up to it?"* to which, I became extremely annoyed and irritated; and began thinking to myself, "How preposterous, is she insane! Here I am looking and feeling like the stay puff woman and you're asking me about washing my hair." Mind you, with my head being so swollen at this time, it appeared as if there was only a small patch of hair on the top of my head that was full of gel; left from the electrodes that were earlier placed throughout. After complaining to my husband, I fell back asleep only to spiral into visualizing all of my organs slowly shrinking and shriveling up like grapes on a vine turning into raisins; one by one.

At the time my body was giving up, shutting down; and experiencing extreme pain when a calm voice began to whisper, beckoning me to go to the light; *"Go to the light Yvonne."*

Regaining consciousness briefly, a nurse standing next to my bed checking my vitals said, *"You must really love your children to continue fighting so hard, but its ok for you to let go and go to the light* honey?" I remember thinking to myself..... *"No, I don't want to go to the light, I'm not ready to go....!"* oddly enough, the entire room at this time seemed to be filled with a very bright soothing golden hue that only I could see. As I asked for the light to be turned off due to its intensity, all who entered my room asked, "What light, there's no light on in here?"

My eldest son, Gregory soon entered the room and said, "Mom it's alright, you can go now if you want too....." and it was then that I knew that I was dying but refused to accept what was happening to me. I simply did not want to leave my children behind however, had I made the decision to do so, somehow I knew that they were going to be alright. Then I was hearing these words again; ***Rollback! Rollback!***

I began to feel my organs expanding; replenishing themselves; slowly plumping up and out, and having a complete feeling of renewal.

Days thereafter, I began to have this feeling of euphoria and a sense of floating in a fog that enveloped me. I floated into the hallway; crossing over into the most beautiful valley and garden—the beauty of it all was extraordinarily breathtaking. I

remember feeling as if something or

someone had compelled me to go in a

certain direction; to a particular room

and window.

As I floated into the room; noticing

this fog like mist all around me. An

elderly female patient's face to the left

of me had a look of bewilderment, but

my attentions were swiftly redirected by

an unknown force of benevolence

summoning me.

Moving closer and closer to this

window, I was unable to control that

which was drawing me; sensing

complete safety. At the same time, I did

not want to let go of these feelings of

absolute.

This force began to beckon me to this

window that I could not turn away from.

There in the distance, appeared

a tiny bright white light about

the size of a pin head; above the

top of the tree line— this light

that seemed so far-off, would

not allow me to turn away.

Unbeknown to me; this would

be the most pivotal moment of

my life and a prelude of what

was to come. As I stared into this

glorious, beautiful, astonishing,

magnificent light; I felt compelled to get

closer.

This bright light began to slowly inch

towards me, growing bigger and

brighter in intensity. There was an

overwhelming need to go to this very

bright light. And just as I thought this

brilliant light would never reach me; it

came at me with such speed and

energetic force, I thought I'd surely be

knocked off my feet.

However, it stopped instantly; just

inches from my face. This magnificent,

beautiful, brilliant white light; brought a

sense of benevolence with an

abundance of love, energy, warmth and

peace so powerful, that I literally felt as

if it had exploded, and flowed

throughout every fiber of my being. A love emanated, of which I had never known; more powerful and a billion times greater than what we know love to be here on earth; a love that transcends all. It would also give me a sense of having a tiny glimpse of God.

This light also brought with it compassion, wisdom, healing and protection; and a voice of calm and reassurance that I would never have to suffer in this way again. And that my life was not yet over. At this moment, I began to beg and plead for it *[the light]* to take me away. The answer given was that it was not my time to go and that I had a mission to fulfill; starting with my family. *"You must go back and rectify the wrongs; tell the world that mankind is destroying itself through hatred and anger; rid yourself of it—get rid of it all!*

Allow the power of forgiveness to take over, and then you will understand. You must learn to love and except Gods love **[God is love, GOD IS LOVE!]** *And if you truly want to know who God is, all you will need is to look within. Just look within yourself and you will find God. [You have nothing to fear my child, nothing to fear! fear has nothing and is nothing but fear itself.] Mankind does not understand that God is universal;*

you are all praying to the same God. It does not matter how you choose to get to God or what path you take, as long as it's the right path. It is your choice! You are all born with the knowledge of right and wrong, good and bad. All that will happen; whether it is good or bad; happens for a reason. There will be many challenges and hurdles placed before you. It is all part of the life lessons God has chosen for you. Which will you *choose? It—is—your choice!"* Then

suddenly this huge brilliant white light

began to slowly radiate down my body;

emitting electrifying warmth that

actually lifted all of the pain, anger and

hatred from my entire body and soul;

granting me total peace and the power

of forgiveness; filling me with God's

love.

The darkest days of my illness no longer

held me in bondage; after being granted

this knowledge of God giving me the answers to questions I had been seeking all along. One of which, not having to question why God would imposed upon me such an illness asking, *"What have I done in my lifetime, O Lord to warrant this type of punishment; a curse such as this?"* Clearly the answer was always right in front of me.

No longer would I have to question the very existence of God, or who God is, or the workings and teachings of God and the universe. No longer would I have to fear anyone or anything. Because the response was instantaneous in disclosing to me through this divine presence; the spoken words that were earlier referenced, of fulfilling a mission. At this point, I immediately looked within myself, as in; literally looking down and peering into my soul (open chest area) as Gods love was being revealed, in the end allowing me to love

myself and find God again.

My heart no longer ached or felt heavy

inside of my chest. The fear of death and

dying was no longer of concern. I now

regard it as being shrouded in eternal

love, peace and comfort.

And once the light reached my feet, it

disappeared, as if a light bulb had blown

out *(blip!)* Leaving what I now know to

be a new person—forever changed for

the better, prepared to heal and face the challenges of this life, this world.

After that, I began gasping for air; taking what I thought to be my last breath.

Upon hearing voices, I tried to turned and walk away, but my legs were like rubber; weak and wobbling. I began to tremble; falling straight back hitting my head on the floor, and hearing a loud cracking sound but feeling no pain. Hospital staffers converged on the room. Immediately I heard questions being asked of me; *"what happened?!?..., How did you get here??..., what is your name?!?"* Then I remember someone saying, *"She's too weak to have gotten out of bed on her own..."* I could not respond. I believe this was when doctors observed me to be possible "postictal" an altered state of consciousness entered after having a seizure. They stated that my eyes were closed and then would open without seeing. Blood pressure was 150/106 and 203/130 during this episode. I gradually responded, woke up and became less "obtunded" (mentally dulled; out of it).

My last memory was of being rolled onto a backboard or blanket and carried away to CCU or ICU. I later learned that I had been admitted one after the other to both units. Additionally, the events may be slightly out of sequence. But again, I am going strictly by what I can recall.

Also, while recounting my experiences to doctors and nurses, they told me that the room in which I was found had a window where I had been standing, but was obscured by a brick wall.

Afterwards, while in ICU, my son Gregory would visit my room several times during the day, staying for hours on end talking, helping to feed, care and watch over me. Even on the days when there was no response; me being in a state of total disconnect with no signs of recognizing him, he stayed right by my side—always a tower of strength, and has always been there for me; of whom I consider to be truly a gift from God...

Once I became totally aware of my situation, I made a promise to be a servant of God asking; *"Heavenly Father, please allow me to live long enough to finish raising my children, and to experience the love of being a grandmother and great-grandmother; and allow your angels of healing and protection to shield me from ever having to go through the same suffering of this*

illness yet again?"

Thus far my wish to be a grandmother

has been granted; fulfilled many times

over, and I have yet to suffer the ordeal

of severe lupus symptoms. I thank you

heavenly father for the blessings.

Critical care unit

In retrospect, this is what also took place while going through my near death experiences; recalled my heart stopped; could no longer breathe; looking over and above my head at the machines monitoring me; stats beeping out of control then flat lining. Hospital staff calling code blue, code blue; sound

of doors slamming closed *(bam bam!).*

I was no longer in my body; watching

as they tried to resuscitate me. After

seeing that I was no longer in my body

floating near the ceiling over my lifeless

body, I exited the room, floating through

the hospital corridors as doctor's race to

my aid. As I hovered and watched from

above; was immediately taken to a place

of darkness and pure evil. Instinctively, I knew this was not a place where I wanted to be. During this time, I and divine beings were in the form of a mass of energy (orbs), being shown different dimensions beginning with what the dark side entails. I asked, *"what is this, where am I?"* a calm strong voice replied; ***"This is pure evil!"*** Then I traveled to a place of void where nothing, only emptiness existed. I was then taken from emptiness into a world in between the heavens and the earth. We all know the saying; "live alone die alone" well to me this was it; where the existence was very lonely and shown what it would be like existing alone with only my thoughts; by myself—I understood. I was then teleported back into this world, and I watched as life carried on as usual without me. I recall there was this invisible wall in between me and the world; could not communicate or move beyond this unseen wall. The next place was of immense light and love which would be my choice of where I'd end up according to how I lived my life here on earth. Switched back to present life in hospital bed; the experience was quite painful upon re-entering my body. I awoke to CCU nurses and a team of technicians monitoring me and asking, *"What is your* name, how many children do you have, who is the president?" to which I responded indignantly, *"Yvonne, three and Clinton of course!"* with tubes, wires and machines all over my body, slipping in and out of consciousness as nurses were going back and forth. Breathing became difficult again (struggling to breathe), extreme sharp shooting pains —heart racing, so much so, that I felt an explosion of my heart was imminent;

then slowing down—flat lining; several times during my thirty-five day stay. This is when visions started to occur of an angel designated specifically to me. Instinctively, I knew this to be much more than visions; taking and showing me the past, present and future events and reviewing my entire life, as though watching a movie reel—what some may refer to as a life review. There was a point when I was made to feel great shame; immeasurable shame for my committed sins that were being placed before me; was forced to relive all; every moment not allowing me to turn away. The sins were what I considered small, but was told, *"The things you consider insignificant, are the things that are most important in Gods eyes."*

They would then go on to reveal much more... I wanted to come back and warn the world of the various disasters about to take place; most of which have already come to pass. But was told I would not be allowed to do so stating, *[You cannot change the course of what is going to take place, you can only cry and pray for the people of this world. All that was shown and told to you will be removed; erased from your memory. In our time all will be revealed; then you will know and understand.]*

They *(angels)* allowed for only a few things to be revealed immediately, such as 911, massive earthquakes, wild fires, droughts, mudslides, and tsunami's; while methodically showing me a map of the world as though it were gradually being dissected and devoured; with only a small portion remaining. As well as, revealing personal / private family information; much of which has also come to pass.

Needless to say, this experience in particular will resonate with me for an eternity.

After fundamentally being given a diagram with the understanding in all that we do here in life, and on earth as being the determining factor of where and how we will live in the afterlife. Not surprisingly, I prefer to take the path that was chosen for me by a higher power.

When referring to the words, *"It is your choice"* meaning; the light or the dark, good or bad—my choice will always be to follow the light, the good; which is God's love.

ANGELIC EXPERIENCE

An angel slowly descended from the night time sky *(heavens)*—oh! What beauty— which seemed like hours as I watched and waited; no longer in my body, suspended above the hospital. The angel stopped in front of me; appearing before me as a huge celestial multi-colored light in the form of a human, with magnificent wings that appeared to span for miles. This divine entity had no gender—appearance was remarkable. We began to discuss why it could not and would not take me. Its duty was to collect the souls of the recently departed —I begged, pleaded and watched as another dearly departed soul was placed upon the angel's chest. As the wings began to envelop this soul, the wing tip gently touched my shoulder, leaving me with a sense and presence of such benevolence; a mighty strength and compassion. The angel telepathically spoke saying, *"I am not allowed to take you; you must stay here; you have a mission to fulfill."* Then ascending to the heavens with lighting speed; leaving a light trail of what appeared to be a dusting of shimmering multi-colored particles of light.

This would continue on over what seemed like several days, the angel ascending and descending, that is. There was no concept of time. Day changing over to night appeared as if watching a movie screen in fast forward motion. The crystal clear blue sky with the whitest of clouds *(the heavens)* zoomed by in all of its beauty and splendor; was glorious. Perhaps, this was in preparation for the darkness to come that would attempt to attack and challenge my mind, body, soul and spirit; testing my very resolve. As the darkness descended, I began clawing my way out of this black hole which was an endless pit of demons snatching bits and pieces of my soul. I fought furiously to struggle and grip each rung of a ladder handed down to me—grasping for dear life, barely managing to hold on; when a strong kind feminine voice urgently called out to me saying, *"You can do it, climb! Don't give up; I will save you! I will carry you on my back, we will climb up together!"* This angel appeared in the guise of a nurse.

As I began to slip, my foot barley touching the bone chilling cold, damp dirt floor; the angel reached down, grabbed and carried me up from the dark cold; deep beneath the hospital basement on her back.

As we climbed to safety the ladder began to transform into body parts comprised of fingers, arms, elbows, legs, knees, toes, heads etc.; connected together by these parts, and realizing that the ladder was my siblings, all fifteen of us with cracks in between each person, essentially symbolizing that there is still much work to be done amongst us; relationship wise.

I awoke from this particular experience being back in my body with no memory of when or how I returned, as a team of medical personnel began asking me questions; my name, age, birth date, what day it was; and holding

up fingers and asking for a count etc.

An affirmation from above that I can truly say without hesitation; there is much more to this life and universe than we will ever comprehend.

THE GREAT ACHIEVEMENT

Learning to walk and talk over again while in the hospital, proved to be a very daunting and arduous task. I attempted to speak and noticed my speech to be in mono tones accompanied with a stammering impediment, added to the fact that I could no longer stand or walk without assistance.

This was something I struggled with for years thereafter; and eventually overcame the majority of. Over time, I regained total use of my right side, as numbness, tingling, burning, and paralysis subsided.

Subsequently, physical therapy was started. As I vaguely recall the drudgery of going to each session; with sheer grit and determination I set out to conquer what appeared in my mind to be an attempt to climb a mountain. Nevertheless, as I completed each task given me, I began feeling more and more of an accomplishment.

The first session proved to be a major struggle, in that, every time I tried to stand up from my wheel chair; my heart and pulse rate would begin to race out of control causing me to feel nauseous and faint. In addition, there was the stress of being forced to go to Physical Therapy and various testing (EMG ,EEG, etc.) in a defective wheel chair with only one foot rest; the very side (right) of which, I had a slight stroke experiencing profound weakness, and needing the additional support, which by the way frustrated me considerably.

However, once notified the matter was swiftly resolved, and I began taking control; focusing on my plight to get back to the task at hand—back on my feet.

Recalling a session when I struggled to get to my feet; the chore of attempting to learn how to walk again, and navigate a flight of stairs was quite challenging, grueling to say the least. Somehow I managed to do it! At this moment I was so proud of what I was doing; taking a few steps and walking up a couple of stairs, WOW! For me this was a major achievement, indeed, considering where I had come from.

TWO WEEK COMA IN HOSPITAL

My room felt a bit stuffy at the time, and I decided to ask the nurse in my room if she could please open the window. She responded in a very harsh tone, *"No, I'm not opening the window for you...."* to which I replied calmly,

"Ok." I then asked if she could please recline my bed for me, and was told without further explanation; that it would not be possible. However, another nurse came in afterwards, and explained that changing my position even slightly would cause my heart and pulse rate to become erratic, an explanation that I could appreciate.

Be that as it may, I was still extremely annoyed with the first response. I then turned my head in the direction of the window; noticing that there were two doves perched on the window sill outside. At this time, I was experiencing difficulty with my vision due to the severe case of conjunctivitis, as well as, massive swelling of eyes and double vision. My eyelids could not close causing pupils to respond as if blinds or shutters were slowly opening and closing, thus requiring multiple applications of eye drops to prevent drying out of eyes.

Glancing over, I could see my reflection in the window, and became distraught and alarmed. Then upon further examination; my entire body seem to be covered with bruises and petechial hemorrhages. I asked for a mirror, and to my dismay, my pupils appeared to be in the shape of a clover leaf along with other abnormalities; leaving me with many questions concerning my overall appearance. No one would answer but much to my relief, I was later informed that my second oldest son, Solomon demanded that comments and questions concerning my appearance be concealed, and further requested that all mirrors be removed from my room; even the tray tables.

My focus turned back on the two white doves, which I could now see clearly; and for some strange reason felt the presence of my grandma and grand-dad. At this moment, I sensed being very much loved, watched over and taken care of; and had a deeply intense understanding that everything was going to be alright. This brought me a measure of immense peace and comfort—was able to relax and go back to sleep.

There would be many times during the worst suffering of my illness, when I would receive visitations from my deceased grandma as I lay paralyzed in fear and extreme pain. I began crying out pleading for her help when she appeared at my bedside. She'd sometimes appear at the foot or the head of my bed depending on what area of my body was experiencing the majority of pain. Placing my head then my feet in her lap, she slowly began stroking and caressing them as warm soothing energy radiated throughout my body, allowing all of the pain to lift and fade away while saying, *"I love you Yvonne, you are going to be ok—this too shall pass,"* which it did. Then suddenly, feelings of total love, peace and comfort surrounded me; allowing me to fall asleep uninterrupted.

SPONTANIOUS HEALING

Soon after, all of my symptoms spontaneously changed, such as;

hemoglobin rising from 7.1 into the 8's getting progressively better. Double vision, severe bruising and broken veins over entire body, bed sore, legs, calves and heel pain miraculously disappeared. By the following day, I became more alert and began asking doctors about my prognosis; attempting to take a more proactive role in my care.

For instance, there was an encouraging moment when my husband entered my room. He awakened me and began excitedly telling me that there were no longer any bruises, blemishes, or broken bulging veins on my legs; in particular the one in the back of my knee. He proceeded to assist in showing me proof by pulling the sheets back and saying, *"Look Yvonne, they're all gone......It's a miracle!"*

Although, the relationship between my husband and I was strained and very much over, he somehow managed to set aside our differences; and pulled it together just long enough to support, and comfort me throughout the majority of my hospital stay. Of which, I love and thank him so very much for stepping up and standing by my side; and will forever be grateful for his attentiveness. From that moment on, and for the remainder of my stay, doctors and staff members referred to me as; *"The miracle woman."*

This brings to mind an incident when doctors requested more blood work; nurses could not find a viable vein; leaving me feeling like a pin cushion and a guinea pig. I then refused to allow anyone else to touch me, forcing a request for a house doctor to be made.

After several unsuccessful attempts by the doctor; a decision was made to place a catheter/shunt into my groin or neck area; procedure was successfully performed. After doing so, the doctor looked down at me saying, *"Oh my God…. you are that miracle woman!*

Do you know it's a miracle that you are still here…?" At this point I was completely speechless.

Thus, leading me to recall another moment when a night nurse by the same name as I, came in as she always did; flashlight in hand, administering meds. At the time, I was up attempting to walk to the bathroom using a tray table to assist me; determined not to use a bed pan. She stopped in her tracks..... Gasping then glanced up at me with a look of astonishment saying, *"You are walking..... How did you get out of bed...? You can't be walking..... But, you can't walk.... You are so tall.... It's a miracle!"* to which I responded sarcastically, *"what are you talking about, I'm standing aren't I?* Just think, the nerve of me standing there weak, wobbly, trembling and out of breath. She sat me down in a chair saying, *"I can't believe this is happening, don't move!"* then turned and literally ran out of my room returning with another nurse; placing me back in bed and cautioning me not to try getting up without calling a nurse for assistance as she walked away repeating over and over again, *"it's a miracle!"*

Being a bit puzzled, I really did not understand at the time the seriousness of the situation with respect in dealing with my condition. Until, upon my release after reviewing my hospital records, the words **"grave condition"** immediately caught my attention. I began to cry an overwhelming cry of relief.

A records clerk noticed my reaction, walked over and asked with thoughtfulness; if I was alright. At that moment, I looked up; thought about it and said, *"thank you for asking, I'm going to be just fine now."*

HOME AFTER COMA

After returning home, and still

trying to process the fact that I was

actually really back home in the flesh.

A sense of possibly being in the spirit world, not being totally connected to this world came over me—I'm sure there are some of you who can relate to what I am trying to express.

However, once entering my house for the first time in over thirty five days, I turned and asked my husband if this was truly happening, me being here, he

responded, *"of course you are here."*

Still unconvinced; standing near the

coat rack, I asked my sons to pinch me

saying, *"I can't believe I'm really here,*

am I really home?" And with a light

pinch while holding on to me they said,

"Yes mom, you really are back home

with us." It soon occurred to me that

this was not just a scene of my life; past

present and future being played out

before me as I had experienced earlier. I

began to recall being told of having the

power to discern. It was setting in that

this—the here and now was my true

reality.

All I wanted after being away for so

long was to sit, and enjoy the comforts

of being back home with my love ones. I

never thought I could be so happy about being home considering how I had left; total dysfunction, chaos and confusion, plus the fact that I was sent home primarily to die. But so much about my life in this short time span had changed. I now had this inner peace where that not anything, or anyone could negatively affect me; causing me to revert back into darkness; and that I was forever protected.

Case in point; while sitting in my living room after my arrival home, my youngest son entered the room and asked, *"Mom why is there a golden light all around your head and face?"* *"And what are those little balls of light flickering all around you?"* My response was that *this is an expression of Gods light, love, healing and angels of protection;* a question that would continue to be asked of me many times over, some from complete strangers. What's more, questions that were considered to be of nuisance, insensitive and even downright rude no longer provoked feelings of discontentment.

My purpose in life was now to concentrate on the power of giving and receiving love and forgiveness; starting with my inner circle. And being eternally grateful for having this second chance at life; a do over, if you will—it doesn't get any better than that! After witnessing what I had gone through, what we had all experienced; it did not matter at the time to my family what condition I returned home in, or how long I had to live. The long and short of it was that I had returned home, back to them; defying all odds. Even with the understanding that there'd be difficult times ahead of us, we managed to move forward, prepared to accept and face whatever challenges lay ahead; and there would be many along the way.

Still, in the end, I have come to the realization, that perhaps this thing was much greater than I, and that I must continue to live my life in accordance to the divine information that was given and shown to me.

MAKING PROGRESS

There were many momentous time when I became aware of my progress upon my arrival back home. However, there was one in particular that impacted me the most. I began to suffering from leg trimmers (restless leg syndrome) that occurred most often during the night. At times, becoming so strong that I'd be awakened from a sound sleep; making it more difficult for me to fall back asleep or walk. Walking was more like shuffling of my feet, due to slight paralysis to my right side that made it more difficult for me to lift them as I took steps. I had a pronounced limp to my right leg. My speech was now stuttered and slurred; which was a result of the lupus related meningitis, including Lupus Cerebritis; causing bouts of confusion, numbness, tingling, burning and jerking sensations in my brain stem; along with other damaging effects that resulted in long and short term memory loss.

Then one day upon awakening, I soon realized that when I would command myself to do certain task such as; pick up your feet when walking, or step over that object (my son lying on the floor at the time), brush your teeth, comb your hair, sit down gently—do not flop down, speak deliberately, etc. I now understood that this was something that had to be done as a form of physical and mental therapy in order to recover from my ordeal; easing the feelings of ambivalence and giving me a sense of empowerment. This revelation was like a breath of fresh air. Speaking of fresh air; the struggle to breathe in and out with ease proved to be quite distressing for me. Awaking to the morning while trying to take in a deep breath; my lungs felt as if they were going to burst—the intense burning felt as if I had inhaled fiberglass. I could actually visualize what was occurring at this time inside of me; seeing all of my blood vessels gorged and expanding with blood while being attacked with ground glass and forced to travel this gauntlet with every gasp.

Then once the air was released, a nice cool feeling began to radiate throughout my lungs with particular attention being directed to my left side; the side that I had experienced the most pain from shrinkage, scarring and pleurisy (best described as inflammation of the pleura; separation of the tissue lining the lungs).

Chemotherapy treatments left me feeling as if I'd been baked crisp, inside and out. I also continued to experience extreme bouts of dry eyes and mouth (Sjogren's Syndrome) this condition occurs when tear and salivary glands fail to function normally due to irregularities; most often forced yawning would sometimes be of help.

Without warning, fingers and toes would start to lose sensation turning cold

(Raynaud's Phenomenon) this occurs when circulation in extremities fail causing numbness with pins and needles sensation. Color changes to blue then white, combined with stiffness, joint aches and pains. A higher dose of steroids was required to suppress the episodes, often resulting in bouts of extreme anxiety and depression.

Most notable of all was the avascular necrosis of both hips *(deterioration of the hip joints due to prescription steroids)* of which, I later had to undergo total bilateral hip replacement surgery, October of 2000.

The surgeon told me that he did not understand how I had managed to get around all of this time saying, *"You should be in a wheelchair, being that one hip had completely collapsed and the other was close to collapsing."* He further stated that upon entering the incision sight while removing the blackened ball socket joint, the ball femur actually disintegrated when placed in his hand. This baffled all who witness and participated in the surgical procedure. They also couldn't understand why I was not experiencing more pain, and requiring more pain medication while in recovery. The recovery nurse further stated, *"Obviously, someone is watching over you.* "At this point, the only words used to describe what was happening were *remarkable, miraculous* and *amazing.*

However, after a long and difficult rehabilitation; healing and resuming my life became paramount. I set out more dedicated and determined to live life to the fullest—regaining what I had lost, and more importantly relying deeply upon; trusting and having faith in my higher power. That which, guided me through a time when I was left to my own devices to make it throughout the day, while on strong medications.

There were times due to poor appetite, when certain medications caused distortions in my mind. For instance: a fast food meal placed before me, still neatly wrapped in an unopened bag, would in an instant have the appearance of being riffled through and crinkled up; then switch back to appearing untouched. And I refused to eat after seeing this. But I also knew that my mind was playing tricks on me. So I contacted my doctor and asked that he cut back the dosages of my medication, which helped me get back to a more normal state.

HELP IS ON THE WAY

One morning I awoke not feeling particularly well; I felt extreme nausea, pain and bloating in my abdomen. At this time I'd only been home from the hospital for a few days. I ask my husband to help me get seated in the recliner, as he was about to leave for the day. The boys had gone to school and I was going to be home alone until they arrive at the end of the day; leaving me vulnerable. Reality was setting in, what was I going to do if an emergency occurred? Well, it didn't take long for me to find out! My abdomen became more distended with unbearable pain, cramping and pressure. I was bleeding internally, and began pleading to God for help in getting to the bathroom. I knew I did not have the strength to stand and walk the distance on my own. Then suddenly I felt what can best be describe as warm energy and powerful hands lifting me out of the chair and helping me walk to the bathroom, but it seemed as if each step had a space under it, producing a floating sensation. Eventually, I reached the commode, and just as I turned and sat down blood began to flow. I literally watched as my abdomen deflated, as if a valve were released. I began to tremble, feeling weak—a sense of peace came over me; the lord had rescued me. I was able to walk gingerly back to my chair and call my husband to inform him of what had happened, he did not come back home until several hours later. Soon after, I went for a colonoscopy and the test results were negative; all appeared to be fine. By this time, I knew that it was only God *(a higher power)*, something of a divine nature that was watching over and taking care of me, walking me through this ordeal; creating a celestial understanding that everything would be alright.

This incident took place as well. My husband was about to leave again early one morning, when I had a bad night with unusual occurrences taking place, such as; an overwhelming bone chilling coldness that enveloped me. So much so, that I had my three boys place two extra comforters over me; and lay over top of and around me to keep me warm. After which, there appeared to be a child size entity that kept entering my room trying to come close to me. One of my sons witnessed this "thing "entering my room and slept on the floor at the foot of my bed to "protect me". The following day, because of these unusual experiences I ask my husband to take me with him, as I did not want to be left alone for concerns of the unexplained. Well, he decided to allow only 15 minutes as he waited outside in the car for me to get ready, after that he was leaving. In that time, I began experiencing things that defied all logic such as; objects disappearing and reappearing, objects (1 gallon water bottles) being in a total state of disarray on the kitchen table, and suddenly stacked neatly side by side on the floor next to the waste basket. Intuitively, I knew this was unnatural; and perceived it to be something of the paranormal. I began again asking for Gods help. At this moment, I was seated and heard a voice say *"Go with him, leave now!"* I began to panic, for I knew that it would be impossible for me to move fast enough to get out in the time allotted me. But again, I felt hands reach underneath me, and carry me almost pushing me towards, and out of the front door at the exact moment that my husband approached the door.

Ultimately, I began wondering; what just happened and why is this happening? I decided to be thankful that I had gotten away from the house. Then later on, as we went throughout the day there were many more strange occurrences while traveling such as; increase in photosensitivity, the intense sun light triggered seizures. They were always preceded by the sound of paper crinkling, a loud clicking, a slow dripping faucet, and clinkering sounds; my body became ridged as I continued to be aware of my surroundings. I began to notice an overwhelming look of fear; even terror on my husband's face. The same look that previously came over him shortly before he'd start to avoid eye contact with me. He suggested notifying my doctor, which I strongly objected to for concerns of being hospitalized again. But, once I realized what was happening I asked him to drive me to the emergency room if this continued to spiral out of control—he agreed. When later asked by my doctor if I was experiencing seizures, I denied ever having any and would have continued denying not wanting to be further hospitalized.

When we arrived back home, my son had been waiting outside for quite some time after school. I noticed his behavior was a bit peculiar. When asked what was wrong he responded, *"Things in the house were disappearing and reappearing in the kitchen."* Basically, giving an exact description of what I had seen and experienced earlier; proof to me that I was not hallucinating or losing my mind. In evidently, this particular revelation cause me to seek out other avenues to better combat whatever crisis I would have to face spiritually, giving me more insight on what I was up against; enabling me to go forth definitely more determined to protect myself and family. Again, I began to ask for divine guidance, which was granted to me by way of receiving special prayers of protection. After which, all strange occurrences ceased to exists.

DIVINE GUIDANCE REVISTED

Not only did I ask for more spiritual guidance, I also received information pertaining to a holistic way of living; obtaining important facts on healing herbs that would help in my recovery; extending well into the future.

I thank the Lord for the wonderful doctors who were willing to work with me emphasizing that whatever you are doing keep on doing it; because it's working! My doctors continued to give words of encouragement.

At last, more confirmation that it is now time for me to resume my life doing more than just existing.

I began to think about the things that brought me innermost peace, contentment and relaxation...Gardening! (Yes, this is something I loved doing) I asked myself,

"Just how are you going to do this?"

Well, I somehow found the strength and

courage to carry on with help and

guidance from my creator. With

tenacity and purpose, I began to slowly

plant my flower gardens again. In the

beginning it was a real struggle and

quite challenging; lifting myself up and

down from my knees; unaware that I

was suffering from deteriorating hip

joints. I often became light-headed and out of breath. Even when leaning my head forward and looking down; my heart began to race and pound inside of my chest causing me to feel faint. I persevered, with the determination of not giving in to my circumstances; as well as, dispensing with all self-pity. My focus was now to continue on taking baby steps, while transitioning towards becoming stronger and healthier.

Incidentally, this would be the most eye-catching flower gardens I've ever grown.

Along with having a mission to feel normal again; by regaining a sense of self-worth and independence, I initiated this by cooking a family dinner; in spite of my limitations. This was something I had longed to do for some time, being that the disease had deprived me of the ability to carry out such familiar task.

But eventually, with absolute willpower I managed to accomplish this all while rolling around in an office chair, carefully taking it one day at a time.

Although it may seem inconsequential, this was one of the ways I chose to start taking my life back; regaining some semblance of independence, while giving me hope and promise that my life would soon be restored back to normal.

SELF HEALING

As I ventured on this journey of

self-healing, with the understanding

that I am being divinely guided every step of the way in what herbs to take that would benefit me the most. I decided that herbal and homeopathic remedies were the way to save and enhance my way of life. After wanting to get away from the conventional medications when being diagnosed with lupus and related heart disease/ heart failure by cardiologists; which by the way is no longer evident. Upon my last cardiology examination, doctors said that my heart was fine. I then sought out to gain as much information as possible on an holistic approach to healing, and began to research everything I could get my hands on concerning homeopathic medications, herbs, vitamins and teas that were eventually taken; and until this day I am currently taking.

Actually, when looking back on my life; the foundation was already instilled by my grandmother who devoted her entire life to spirituality and healthy living. I also credit her with giving me a start in the knowledge of herbs and their healing properties during the early seventies ultimately, preparing me for my future in overall healing of the mental and physical body.

More importantly, I knew that in time I would have to find something to reverse the damaging side effects from medications such as; steroids, chemo, radiation etc., and the ravages of the disease itself; as a result leading me to the alternatives. Some of the conventional drugs actually exacerbated my condition; leaving me with no choice other than to seek out homeopathic herbs and meds to promote healing.

Therefore, I am more than willing to divulge this information to whoever thinks it will help to benefit their lives. And these are the homeopathic medicinal aids that have allowed me to live a more normal life.

✓ One of the first herbs taken was Taheebo tea *(Pau'D Arco)* tree bark. I decided to take this herb after being diagnosed with

Hemangiomas of the Liver and Uterine Fibroids. This particular herbal remedy is known to shrink and dissolve tumors. After consuming this tea daily for more than a month; upon my next visit to my doctors, they found the liver tumors to have shrunk and stopped growing. In addition, the fibroids were also gone which were diagnosed prior as being massive. Incidentally, this herb and also Bromelain at least 1500mg per day with 3 papain tabs per day helps with bloating, weight loss, indigestion and the overall distortion of appearance that is associated with steroid use. Having lost my gallbladder years earlier, Bromelain was quite beneficial in helping with digestion.

✓ Other herbs and vitamins taken were gotu kola, alpha lapoic acid, holy thistle (blessed thistle) and neuro ps for brain/memory enhancement which help me after suffering brain damage sustained during my two week coma. The burning, jerking and tingling sensation to my brain stem took more than a year, gradually subsiding along with restless leg syndrome upon taking these supplements.

✓ Immune boosting vitamins and herbs such as; Cod Liver Oil, Oil of Oregano, Colostrum, Olive Leaf, Red Clover Blossom,

Vitamin C, Calcium w/ D,E,B6, B12, multi vitamins, Iron tabs.

✓ Larrea: helps kill viruses if taken at the onset. I found this to be highly effective when I contracted a cold or virus.

✓ Vitamins and herbs for skin health:

Alpha Lopoic Acid (helps fight cell damage), Gotu Kola, Pine Bark Extract, Plantain Leaf, Borage and Burdock help in treating severe skin conditions, hair loss, nerve health and joint stiffness. Hydrolyzed collagen liquid protein (strengthens & repairs collagen tissue, skin, blood vessels & connective tissue). This liquid protein will definitely benefit anyone diagnosed with all types of arthritis, joint aches and pains; and has been a life saver greatly benefitting me overall in many ways since 1996; also helping me to get a more restful night's sleep when taken at bedtime.

✓ Liquid extract such as: Silymarin Milk Thistle helps to detoxify the liver and helped to repair the damage caused by chemo, radiation, steroids and other prescription medications that proved to have a toxic effect on my system.

✓ Hawthorn berry helps to regulate blood pressure and helps with heart health. Other heart health herbs taken were *Astragalus Root*: Excellent energizer and immune system stimulant, also fights viral infections and helps heart condition; strengthening the heart. Can benefit diseases of lungs and kidneys as well. Aconite, passion flower, blessed thistle (holy thistle) is an excellent stimulant tonic for heart and stomach. Also strengthens memory by circulating oxygen to brain, and is good for gas, heartburn and stomach problems. Blessed thistle was excellent in treating my lungs, kidneys and liver; cleanses blood.

✓ For lung health I took coltsfoot (helps in removing chest phlegm), pennyroyal (benefits chest and lungs). Borage is also an anti-inflammatory, when used as a tea helped to improve and repair lung damage inflicted by the lupus disease. I no longer suffer from bouts of pleurisy or pneumonia since taking these combined herbs.

✓ Feverfew: helps with migraines, restores liver to normal function and reduces joint inflammation.

✓ Chamomile flower: excellent for overall calming of nervous system. Helped to reduce anxiety attacks.

✓ Nettle: helps the lungs, skin, kidneys and blood. I also found it to reverse graying of hair. Good for fevers and colds.

✓ White oak bark: helps to restore circulation. This was very helpful in treating my DVT and Reynaud's phenomenon, in addition to placing my hands in very warm water which helped in restoring circulation. Upon taking this herb my symptoms began to dissipate.

✓ Myrrh: cleans colon and helps to regulate the digestive system. Also helps to improve sinus problems while benefitting your body's entire system. Fibromyalgia syndrome, TMJ and abdominal ulcers disappeared after taking this herb.

✓ Aloe Vera juice and gel: taken initially to boost immune system, also helped with arthritis and stomach problems.

✓ Nephritis of the kidneys (renal failure): lecithin is what was initially taken to help cleanse and purify my kidneys. Uva- ursi Leaf, barberry and birch bark helped with bladder and kidney infections.

✓ Burdock root and red clover: removes toxins from body (blood purifier) very beneficial to entire system. Also helps with skin problems.

✓ Damiana: helped with reducing menopausal symptoms.

✓ Sciatica: after suffering for many years from sciatica, I began taking homeopathic drops called sciatica, and have not had a single episode in more than twelve years.

✓ Plantain Leaf: used for chronic skin problems.

✓ Kombucha: This herb helped to detoxify and energize my body. Also helps to benefit your entire body's system.

✓ DMSO: One eight to one quarter teaspoon of this substance daily in a half glass of water for up to two weeks at a time, along with one tsp of food grade oxy peroxide is what I began to take when I received lab reports of near perfect, and perfect kidney function, plus that my lupus was now deemed to be inactive; leaving me to say with great certainty that all of my symptoms were significantly helped and even diminished after using these substances. The only downside was the DMSO odor.

✓ Pine bark extract and horsetail: After experiencing loosening of my teeth, and severe gum/ tooth pain; I contemplated having all of my teeth removed until I found these two herbs. Horsetail helps the glandular system and is also good for hair, nails, teeth, eyes, nose, and throat. Pine bark helped to reduce inflammation and pain. Of which I found to be the perfect solution. And with the combined use over time of taking all of what I've listed as medicinal aids; I no longer had to endure the tremendous discomforts of lupus symptoms.

Since taking these herbal and homeopathic supplements my emergency visits seeking medical attention have greatly diminished. I have not been hospitalized since early 2000's for lupus related ailments.

DIET AND EXERCISE

Modification of diet played a significant role in treatment of this disease. I decided to invest in a juicer and began drinking vegetable/fruit juice daily. This generally helped to elevate my energy level.

But there were certain foods I had to avoid such as; alfalfa sprouts, bean sprouts, chickpeas peas, soybeans, mushrooms and legumes. Also, certain citrus such as; oranges, grapefruit and especially mangos, avocados and kiwi (used the process of elimination) this is with most foods. Nuts such as; peanuts, brazil, almonds, cashews, pistachio, pecans and smoked nuts. White rice, white flour and refined sugars were very problematic. Dairy products such as milk, orange juice, cheddar cheeses, etc. and smoked foods (meats, cheeses, fish etc.)

Fish such as; salmon, shellfish, shrimp, crab, lobster etc., and certain oils such as; safflower and peanut oil, as they were sure to aggravate my condition by producing joint aches/pains, muscle and joint stiffness, nausea, headaches and causing additional flare ups.

Proper nutrition is essential to maintaining your health, again use the process of elimination in order to determine which foods your body can best tolerate.

Stay active while getting the proper exercise and rest. Do not over exert yourself as I did early on. There was a time prior to being diagnosed, when I walked up to four miles a day, sometimes twice a day to stay fit. During this time, I started to experience extreme muscle weakness, burning joints and diarrhea shortly after each workout. Only to be informed later that I was experiencing "muscle wasting." Therefore, it is crucial to avoid participating in too much strenuous activity; causing over use of muscles. Minimize your workouts, but stay consistent.

Also keep in mind that most individual cases of lupus are different. Some have more or less symptoms than others. My case was very unusual, in that, I exhibited criteria associated with all types of lupus (systemic, discoid and drug-induced).

My doctor at one point even suggested that I'd make a great case study, but I totally rejected the thought of such a thing. In my mind this would have been admitting to defeat, which I could not even fathom at this time.

On the other hand, it made perfect sense from a medical perspective; provided that cases thereafter would have vastly benefitted given my information.

So with that being said, whatever you're diagnosed with, make sure to stay under close medical supervision.

Hopefully, you will be fortunate enough to find doctors that will work collectively, and agree with the combined use of conventional and homeopathic treatments and cures as I have. Take a stand, and begin to properly manage your illness.

THE POWER OF LOVE AND SUPPORT

The thing I can't stress enough is that you must surround yourself with a positive support system; people who will believe in you and helping you to heal..... Here's a perfect example of how the love, support and caring of loved ones can greatly influence a situation; and why my love will forever extend deeply in appreciation to all who supported and stood by me when I needed them the most; especially my children.

My children were by my side daily for the entire time I was hospitalized. There were mornings when I'd awake to a room filled with my children, their friends and classmates visiting prior to the start of school or work; surrounding my bed and reciting prayers and scriptures. This helped to encourage me in my fight to strive and get well. Then too, throughout my entire stay it was the love and concern shown by my mom via phone that helped to sustain me. Just having the sound of her sweet voice expressing her beliefs that everything was going to be alright; while conveying messages that all of my family members and friends were praying for me made a considerable difference. This in spite of the fact that mom was in no condition to travel due to my father's recent passing; she somehow managed to stay in constant contact with me and my doctor, pleading for him to do what he possibly could to save my life. She then continued on to send words of encouragement and reassurance that all would be ok.

However, with hindsight on this whole ordeal, I often wondered why we; meaning husband, children and I had to go through this suffering virtually alone physically. The answer was that must be this was how it was meant to be. It was God's will that we travel this journey alone together; in light of the deep divide that we allowed amongst us. Therefore, there were valuable lessons yet to be learned about the true meaning of family, and this was the only way to convey that message.

In relation to having a continual strong supportive foundation, I am reminded of past conversations that I had with one of my physicians. Often, during my darkest moments, I thought about how this doctor made me feel totally at ease. As though, there were a deep connection between us; and that I could be quite open and candid with her. She

presented herself as very personable,

dedicated, and devoted and caring to

her profession, and to me the patient—

sentiments I extend to nearly all of my

doctors. Over the years, she would go

on to give me advice ranging from

medical to personal information that I

would use in the years to come. The

story that stands out in my memory

most vividly is when she spoke of going

on a spiritual pilgrimage, which involved

walking up a mountain with her husband

and a vast group of people with various

medical conditions; while battling

cancer. She went on to explain how

there were times when she thought she

would never make it to the top; due to

her extreme weakened state. But with

prayer and the determination to live,

she managed to get to the top of the

mountain, stating that, *"my trust and*

faith in God is why I am standing here

before you today". She also went on to

discourage me from taking

recommended chemotherapy

treatments when first diagnosed with

lupus saying, *"It will destroy your body,*

do not do what I did. Prayer is also what

is going to help you. Go home and

prepare a sacred room in your house.

Get on your knees and pray there

together with your family, ask for

strength and guidance." This to me was the soundest advice given early on, which I was more than willing to follow, along with continuing on with medical care. Her words became an inspiration for what I was about to face, by giving me hope and direction, for which I am so very grateful that our paths crossed when they did. These words provided me with a constant reminder of how very important family, life and living is.

TAKING CONTROL

Make an effort to inject a little humor into your life along with music. Learn to laugh even if you can't do anything but listen to something you find amusing, because both can actually be quite beneficial; therapeutic and healing.

For a short period of time, I found myself losing touch with both genres that I held so near and dear to my heart. After a while, I made a decision to dig deep down inside channeling my inner spirit; and fought hard to recapture the love from deep within.

In fact, I found that when relying on my love of music and humor; even joking about my then catlike appearance and mimicking *"meow!"* It made the symptoms and disfigurements from the disease easier to except and get through.

Quick story; alone one day after being home for several weeks; a UPS delivery arrived. I was hesitant to go to the door because of my unsightly appearance, but decided to answer it any way.

Upon opening the door, the gentleman (my regular carrier) gasped in shock, taking a couple of steps back with a look of complete terror; anxiously waiting as I signed. Speechless, he abruptly turned and all but ran back to his truck; jumping in and speeding off.

After closing my door, I turned to see myself in the mirror (Whew!) and instantly knew why he reacted in such a manner. For the first time since being home, I recognized that my appearance was skeletal in nature (emaciated) with protruding blood shot eyes and patches of hair on my head; a drastic change from how I use to look. In spite of this, I nearly fell over in laughter in light of what had just happened.

Over time, a complete recovery was soon to follow; regaining weight as swelling gradually disappeared, as well as, growing back a healthy thick head of hair; returning back to normal. This was a classic example of choosing to find humor in my circumstance, rather than wallowing in self-pity and falling into a state of depression. And still to this day, I can look back on this moment and have a good laugh.

Therefore, always remember that laughter is truly the best medicine, and good for the soul. Please just keep in mind that these maladies may only be temporary. Embrace and except what is transpiring in your life. Begin to take charge with the mindset of not settling in no uncertain terms to doom and disappointment; and do not give in to your circumstance. Begin to make life and living your life a priority.

For instance, once I learned that I was one of only three worldwide to survive going through to the end stages of lupus; the disease settling in my brain, I knew that there would not be anything that I could not overcome.

This has been the motivating factor leading me to help others, in hopes that you too will consider yourself to be a survivor and not a victim.

This is imperative!!!!! Learn to love yourself; love you first and only then will you be able to move forward in helping others as well. Furthermore, begin to rid yourself of all that is toxic in your life; mainly anything that is stress related. Because once I got rid of the toxic people/person in my life, my health turned completely around; plus the fact that I have a strong spiritual foundation/ support system. In fact, after many years of almost complete isolation, I finally found the courage to take back control of my life. The first step was in becoming liberated; through seeking therapy for me and my children. Then after finally being diagnosed with PTSD (post-traumatic stress disorder), which was a direct result of spousal abuse and the majority of my stress, ultimately a name was now attached to what had caused such trauma and suffering in the past.

Finally last but not least; the termination of my marriage. Unfortunately this was long in coming and necessary. However, this I can attribute to my present state of remission. So my message to you is that if I survived this journey into and through lupus, you can too. All that you will need is to put total trust and faith in God, your higher power. Take the approach to always expect the unexpected; allow this to be your guide, and never let anyone or anything get in your way, especially when it infringes upon your survival as a human being.

Eventually, I joined self-help support groups that were instrumental in helping to turn my life around. With the intervention of these organizations, I took the necessary steps that enabled me to go back to school; enrolling in and completing college courses that has helped to advance my ambitions towards rebuilding my life and future. I cannot express enough the importance of giving me back my confidence and self-esteem that I had lost and so desperately needed. Therefore, I'd like to thank all of you for your support. Sending lots of love, you all know who you are....I wish you well and will never forget you; we were team! As for my three chief mentors; Robin, Eve and

Mary Ann; Thank you! Thank you! Thank you from the depths of my heart! May God forever bless you for saving and changing lives!!!!!

Overall, the experience of embracing my illness has made a tremendous difference in how I will go forth living my life. Equipped with the knowledge that life's too short to be consumed with negativity; I plan to focus on and allow only the positive aspects of life to influence and guide me by living totally in the moment; making me a stronger woman/person. And you must learn to do the same. So therefore, when obstacles come your way, you'll have the will to triumph over them as I continue to do. For this reason, I am revealing my story in hopes of representing my contribution to the

healing of this world.

I wish you healing light and

love.

Yvonne's ACKNOWLEGEMENTS

First and foremost, I'd like to thank my heavenly father; God almighty for allowing me to live another day, and for the blessings that you have bestowed upon us. And ask that you continue to send your white light all around us filled with your God given love, peace, compassion, healing and protection.

Gregory and Gigi (son & daughter) for your continuous show of love, support and dedication; I send an abundance of love and gratitude. I also credit you with encouraging me to persevere in spite of the inconceivable obstacles that lay ahead. You made it all possible, in the fact that you have always been there for me; even in the worst of times, which speaks volumes. I cannot begin to express enough how very much I love and appreciate you both for all that you have done for me over the years. Thank you for never wavering my eternal love....

Gregory and Aaron (my sons) thank you for your love, support and prayers when I needed them most. You all stood steadfast by my side helping me to heal, and giving me the confidence to survive this ordeal;

virtually willing me to live. Your mere presence afforded me the strength to continue the fight, which I did and for this I am forever grateful, with my love being everlasting. Thank you again, and I love you truly.

To my estranged son Solomon; though you broke my heart, I still pray that you would someday find your path back to God and our family. It was difficult to forgive you for your hurtful and shameful actions however, at the insistence and council of your brother and sister in-law (Gregory & Gigi), I came to realize that you need my love more than ever. I know that someday you will find peace and set aside the confusion and anger which has consumed and corrupted your soul. You like your brothers, are the best hope for the future and be mindful that you are raising future Lightner women. Protect them from harm and see to it that they never accept that domestic violence of any kind is acceptable. Respect their mother and you will find that peace which you seek. Most importantly embrace who you are. No matter how you chose to lead your life, you will not be judged for being who you truly are. Your struggle began very early in life and all I want is for you to be happy no matter who and how you chose to love. Know that when I removed you from my life you it had nothing to do with your alternative lifestyle.

Thank you so very much to my sister Cathy for your constant support of me and my family throughout. The fact that you were able to capture, and illustrate in your paintings the exact scenes of my divine experience before ever being told was astounding, as well as, God sent. I'd like you to know that our bond is forever; and will never be broken. You were the confidant that I deeply relied on when the road became too rough; by stepping up and keeping me spiritually grounded. It is mostly for this I love you dearly.

Here's to sending loads of love to each and every one of my siblings and their families for embracing me with your love, support, understanding and prayers when I reached out to you. This also speaks to extended family as well. Thank you, thank you, and thank you!

To all of my very precious grandchildren, all thirteen of you; Savion, Giana, Gilina, Gevont, Giavonna, Alicia, Yvonne, Shane, Seth, Micaila, Leah, Aaron and Isaac you have given me so very much unconditional love, as well as, shown me how to love. You mean the world to me, which makes life even more precious than you will ever know. Lots of love, hugs and kisses!

Much love to you Odetta and Cheryl for your true friendship of love, support and many words of encouragement. You stood by me through all of the insanity, and I sincerely appreciate and thank you.

I'd also like to take a moment to extend a personal thank you to the hospital staff and doctors who expressed genuine concern in caring for me and my family during my convalescence.

A special thank you to nurse Donna for not only going above and beyond the call of duty, but also serving as a therapist of sorts. Allowing me to pour out my inner most personal feelings and just being a good listener; providing me with a very cathartic experience.

Thank you, Dr. Gabel, Dr. Gopal and Dr. Otrakji and staff for your constant care, service, devotion and support throughout the years. I send to you all an abundance of gratitude. And you will forever be in my thoughts and prayers.

With great appreciation, Dr. Mary and staff of the Parker clinic for your care and service that also reached above and beyond the call of duty. You were there for me when I was at my lowest point financially. Thank you so very much for making medical care and treatments attainable.

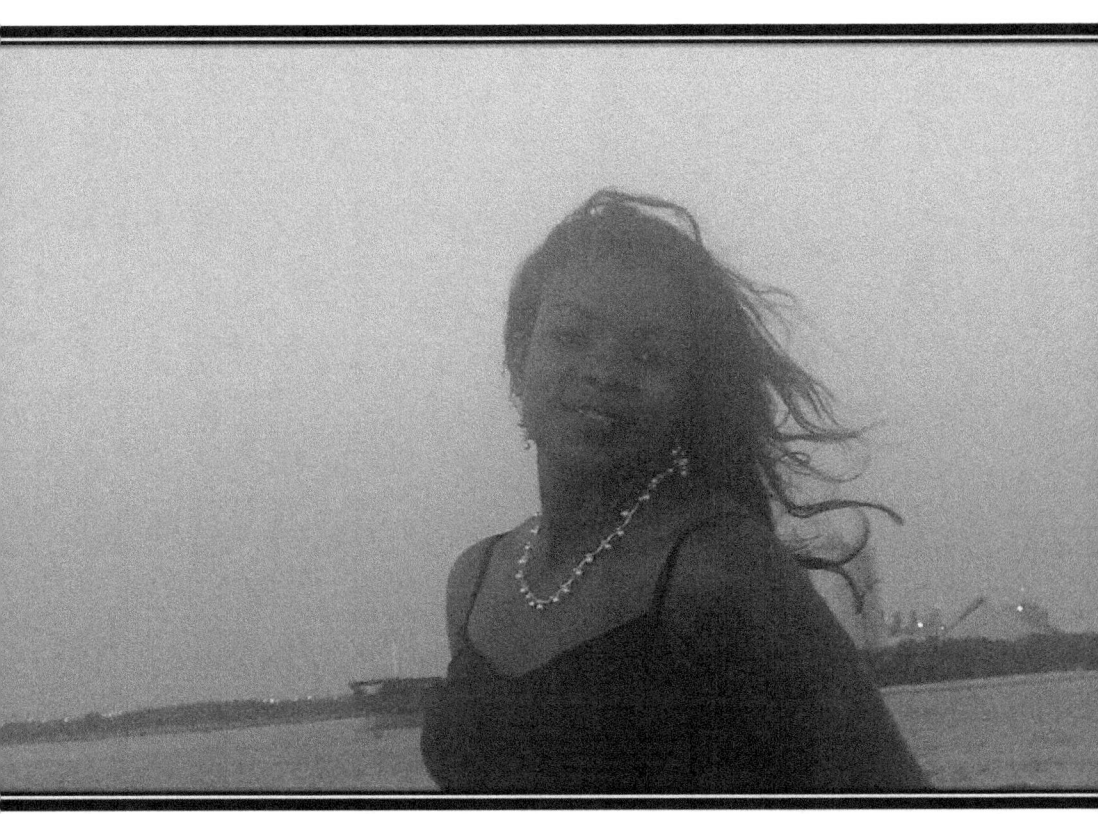

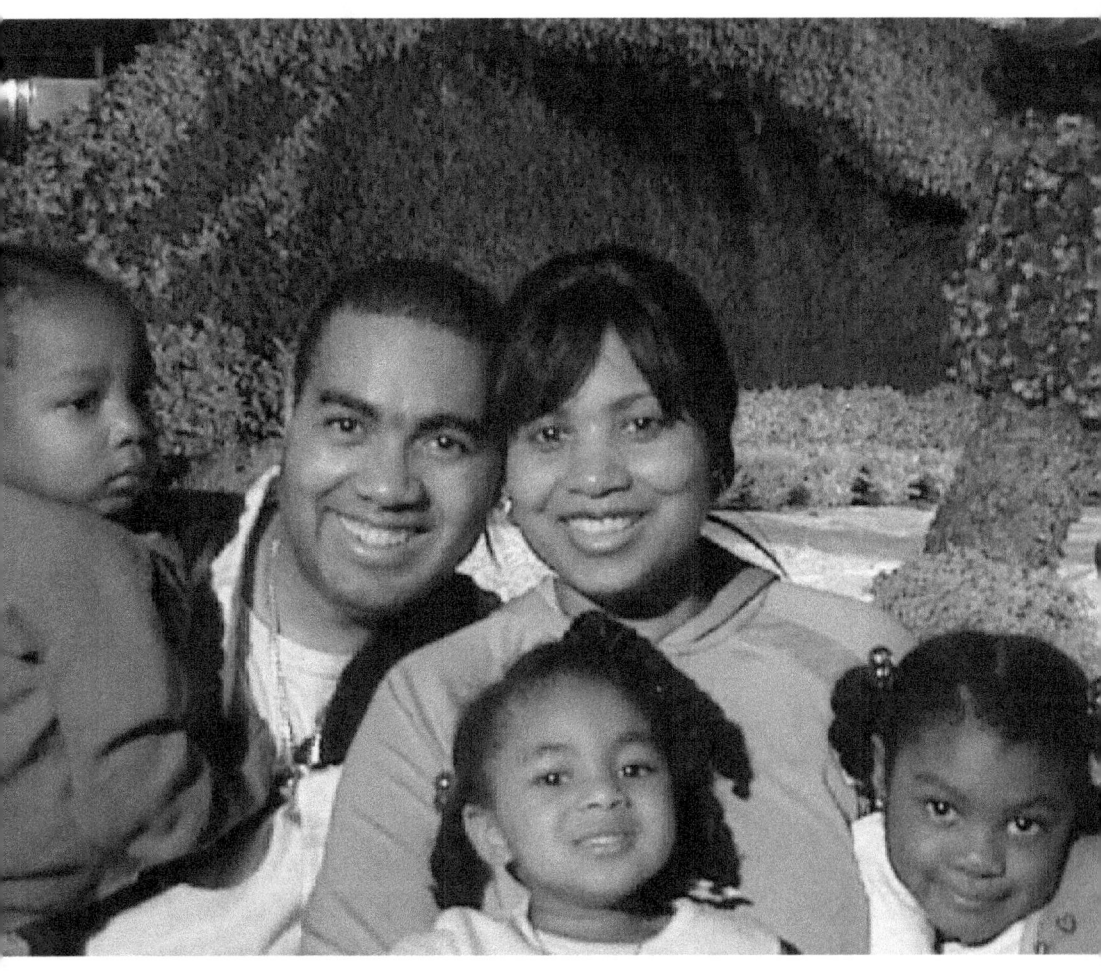

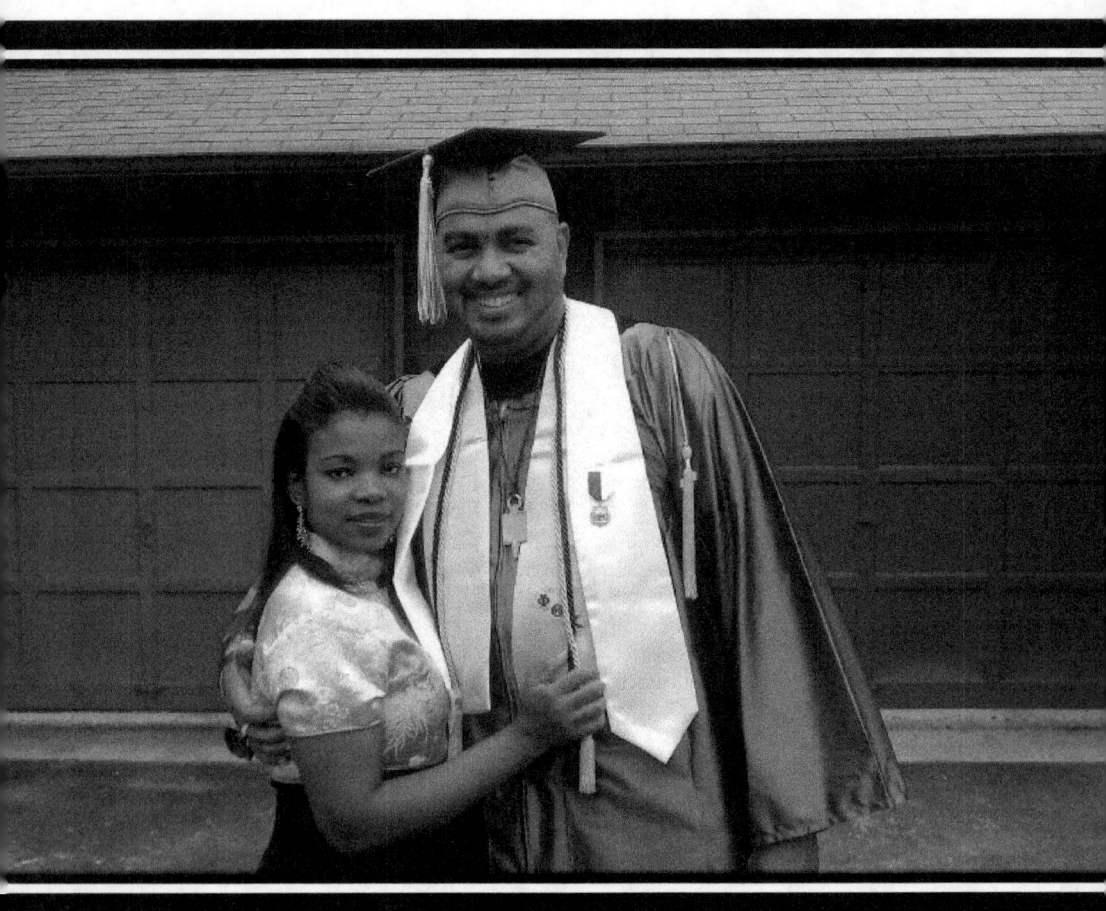

COMMENTARY

Author Gregory T. Lightner Jr.

"_____ is sick all the time… she (or he) always has something wrong with them!! It's no big deal."

Inclosing, I would like to address everyone who has a loved one who may be far away or out of touch for some reason or another. The most important lesson that I have learned is how death affects people differently. It's never a good idea to wait until someone is near the end of their life to say you love them or show concern. If you have an opportunity to see them now don't make excuses or take them for granted. Those who have Lupus suffer chronically, and there is no cure. Many times Lupus patients are regarded in the following manner, "_____ is sick all the time; she (or he) always has something wrong

it no big deal." This statement is often attributed to people

who don't understand the disease. The fact is things can

go bad in a hurry for Lupus patients. Speaking from

experience, my mother made many calls to friends &

family that went unreturned over the last years of her life.

Invitations to come visit were ignored or disregarded all

together. My mother knew that her time was short for her

life and was reaching out. Similarly, I reached out to

friends and family as well and many were able to visit or

called regularly and have good lasting memories while she

was still vibrant and able to enjoy them. It was

disappointing that many waited until my mother was no

longer coherent(Literally waited to the day before she

passed) and wanted me to put the phone to her ear so

they could say goodbye to what had become a dying

broken shell. The worst thing to do is wait until the very end of a person's life to become concerned. This can often be seen as a failure to be considerate of the person & family whom are caring for that person. The reality is that you will face hostility & anger in the short term from those who are the immediate caregivers. Long term resentment may also follow if you cannot find a way to apologize to those whom you have inadvertently damaged. Being a caregiver is not an easy task and it is unreasonable to expect that they are not under tremendous stress. Failure to recognize this will absolutely create interpersonal conflicts that can be very difficult and in some cases impossible to overcome.

As my mother's most vocal supporter I sometimes felt overwhelmed at the task at hand. I was often the only *buffer between those people whom only wanted to cause my mother pain and shorten her life by applying stress. It was during this time however, that I can truly say that I was challenged to reach potential that I use to only dream of. In the last few years I was able to be a point of joy for my mother as she constantly was able to be present each and every moment with us. Though she is no longer earthbound, her ethics, morals and spirit live on in in her descendants. My children had the honor of knowing that they were loved by Grandma Yvonne and were with her when she drew her last breath.*